The Prescription for a
Lifetime of Great Health

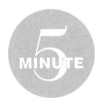

THE Doctors

5 MINUTE

Health
Fixes

The Prescription for a
Lifetime of Great Health

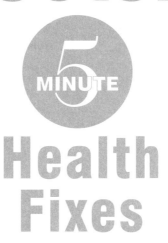

THE Doctors

5 MINUTE

Health
Fixes

THE DOCTORS with Mariska van Aalst

RODALE

Library of Congress Cataloging-in-Publication Data
The doctors 5-minute health fixes : the prescription for a lifetime of great health / the doctors with
Mariska van Aalst.
    p.   cm.
  Includes bibliographical references.
  ISBN-13   978–1–60529–326–4 hardcover
  ISBN-10   1–60529–326–1 hardcover
  1. Health—Popular works.   I. Aalst, Mariska van.   II. Title: Doctors five-minute health fixes.
RA776.D63 2010
613—dc22   2010026692

Distributed to the trade by Macmillan
2   4   6   8   10   9   7   5   3   1   hardcover

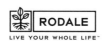

We inspire and enable people to improve their lives and the world around them

For more of our products visit **rodalestore.com** or call 800-848-4735

The Doctors wants to dedicate this book to all the people who are facing some of life's most challenging health issues and to those who are taking the necessary steps to create a healthier lifestyle. *The Doctors,* its experts, and its production team are committed to bringing our viewers the latest medical information and tools for healthier living.

Contents

The Doctors Are On Call— For You

What is the one truly irreplaceable resource? Time.

We all want more time:

- more time to ourselves

- more time to sleep

- more time to develop our talents

- more time to travel, to experience new things

- more time with our spouses or significant others

- more time with our kids or grandkids

- more time to enjoy our lives

With an eye toward saving time, we've created machines to do our work for us. Think of all the time-saving machines we've developed over the past 100 years.

Instead of washing our clothes by hand, wringing them out, hanging them up on the line, taking them down from the line, ironing them with an iron heated over a fire (which was built by hand), what do we do?

We put our clothes into a box and press a button. Then we put them into another box and press another button. (Can't get around that folding, though.)

And think about our food. Instead of tilling the soil and growing our food, picking out the weeds every day, chasing down and slaughtering our dinner, plucking feathers, gutting deer, climbing trees or crawling through vines, chopping and slicing and canning, we do this:

We toss a package into a box, close the door, and press a button.

For most of us, all of this time "saved" is not translating into time spent doing things that improve our lives. With the time we save by nuking a frozen dinner or e-mailing a colleague who is 20 feet away, we're more likely to . . . well, eat junk food and sit on our butts.

And as we squander that time, we're also squandering our health. In the process of using more of these time-saving measures to save ourselves effort, we've been robbing our bodies of the exercise they used to get and the whole, fresh foods that we used to nourish them with. In a way, all those time-saving tools might actually be *stealing* time from us—because we may be dying sooner.

Well, no more! We're here to show you how you can create time. How you may be able to add 2, 4, 10, 20 years to your life—good years, active years. Fun years.

And you're going to do it starting today. Starting right now. Because we're going to show you something amazing: You only really need 5 minutes to make a change that lasts a lifetime.

We're Not Only Doctors, We Play Them on TV

Every weekday since September 2008, we've come into homes all over America to help you make sense of the conflicting medical information that comes at you from so many sources. We debate each other and share our thoughts about the biggest health headlines, the most controversial new procedures, and the embarrassing questions that people are scared to ask their own doctors. We take that information and turn it into positive solutions that impact viewers' lives.

If you've seen the show, you know we serve up our health information with a little bit of sass and a lot of science. Hey, we're not only doctors, we're also guinea pigs. From herbal teas to exercise machines to avocado facials, we love to try out as many of the cures we cover as possible—sometimes to very surprising, silly, or even (when we're feeling brave) gross effect. And if we can have a chuckle in the process, all the better. Laughter is the best medicine, right?

But while we like to have fun, we also take our jobs very seriously: We want to help everyone in the world—including you!—enjoy better health. We doctors can literally be lifesavers—but the only person who can *keep* you healthy is *you*. You have to make health a priority—and one of the best ways to keep it that way is to make it fun. That's where we come in. We are:

Dr. Travis Stork, an emergency room doctor who plays a mean game of hoops (if he does say so himself). He taps into his experience treating thousands of critical and life-threatening medical problems to help you determine important health choices to make every day

Dr. Lisa Masterson, an obstetrician and gynecologist who can't live without her heels and helps women stay sexy and strong so they can live happy and healthy lives and empowers women of all ages at every stage of their lives

Dr. Jim Sears, a pediatrician who is always game to try the wackiest, scariest, and most disgusting—hello, Neti pot!—remedies with a goofy good humor that makes his little patients (and their parents) love him

Dr. Drew Ordon, a plastic and reconstructive surgeon who gets jazzed by doing groundbreaking treatments on the air and who shows us that radiant beauty and good skin are well within the grasp of every woman and man in America, with or without plastic surgery

Between the four of us, we've received thousands of letters and e-mails from viewers all over the country. And we love that some viewers can come on the show to share their stories and ask for advice. Given the time constraint, however, we can only help so many people. Often, we find ourselves at the end of the hour saying, "Man, I wish we could have talked longer about that," or "I hope we answered that question fully." It's the quintessential 21st-century dilemma: There's just never enough time!

Yet when we step back and consider those e-mails and letters and stories together, we see that, essentially, they generally boil down to the same question:

"How can I enjoy my life and my health and stick around more years?"

Now, no matter how much advice and information we can share in an hour of television, tackling that question is still a tall order. Which is why we decided to write this book.

In your hands, you hold the information you need to help answer that question. We've developed solutions so simple, so straightforward, that you can start *today*, in just 5 minutes.

Sound too good to be true? We thought it might. But believe us: You're going to be stunned by what we found.

What *Does* Help Us Live Longer—And Better?

As medical professionals, we always begin with science. We draw all of our recommendations, both on the show and in our own practices, from a methodology doctors call evidence-based medicine. Simply put, we combine our clinical experience with the most credible scientific information available to make the best possible recommendations to our patients.

With this approach to inspire us, we formulated a plan for this book: What aspects of health are the most critical to long-term vitality? Keeping in mind that, in today's crazy, time-crunched world, no one can do it all, what are the areas the average person can focus on to help safeguard his or her long-term health?

To find the answers, we looked at many dozens of studies examining millions of people throughout the world. We sought to isolate the aspects of health that most often corresponded with long-term vitality. And what we found was actually very straightforward: If we focus our efforts on 10 key areas of health, we can live longer, more vital lives.

As busy professionals ourselves—we're all practicing doctors with active personal lives and volunteer duties, in addition to spending a few days a week taping the show—we knew that readers weren't going to sign up for any inflexible, time-consuming program. So we crafted the advice in this book to fit into the typical all-too-crazy life—instead of asking you to reengineer your life to fit the program, we've engineered the book so that it truly fits you, your needs, your life.

If you've watched the show, you know we are always up for a challenge—especially when we're challenging each other! So we set a goal for ourselves: To offer only tips that can have the *maximum* impact in the *minimum* amount of time. Using 5 minutes as the time limit for most of the fixes we would suggest—because, c'mon, we can do anything for 5 minutes, right?—we delved into the research in all of the relevant fields, gathering together the most efficient ways to enhance your health and potentially extend your life starting *right now*.

Sounds good, right? Maybe too good?

"C'mon, Doctors," you might be thinking. "That's a bit of a stretch."

How can we possibly make that claim—that you may actually extend your life with a change that takes just 5 minutes?

Well, try this on:

- One Italian study found that if you eat a small piece of dark chocolate every day for 15 days, you could shave 6 points off your blood pressure and significantly enhance your body's insulin response, a key to preventing diabetes
- Use a paper filter in your drip coffeemaker instead of using a gold one or drinking French press coffee and you could decrease your cholesterol by 8 percent, reducing your risk of heart disease
- Floss your teeth in the morning for 30 seconds to help prevent periodontal infections that raise the risk for heart disease, diabetes, and respiratory diseases—possibly adding 6.4 years to your life
- Have sex at least once a week and cut your risk of erectile dysfunction by 200 percent. Bump that up to two or three times a week, and you decrease your risk of heart attack or stroke by 50 percent—and add up to 8 years to your life.

How is it possible that such small things can have such big effects? (Guys, when we say small, don't get paranoid—we're obviously not talking about sex here.) The human body is an incredibly resilient, thriving machine that *wants* to be healthy. Your body just needs you to put in a bit of effort here and there and it will do the rest.

Now, consider that the suggestions above are among the easiest "fixes" you can make. (We sincerely doubt, for example, that any guy is going to fight us on the sex thing—especially Dr. Jim.) But imagine what can happen if you add, say, 5 extra minutes of walking the dog each time you take Fido outside? Or if you decide you're going to stop worrying so much or actually take your vacation this year? Combined, changes like these could reap gains of several years, not just weeks or months.

Now multiply these changes by the hundreds of suggestions and tips packed into this book. You could be on your way to 2, 5, 10, even 13 or 16 extra years of life—simply by making a few of these small changes every day.

But adding years to your life is not the only benefit—not by far. Consider the quality of the life you'll add to those years. You'll be better able to play with your kids and your grandkids. You'll be able to scale those staircases—and then, possibly, a mountain or two. You might go from exercising with an aerobics DVD to taking tango lessons. You might move from a stationary bike to a road bike to a racing bike—who knows what you'll do with your increased energy, strength, and vitality?

We know one thing you'll do with it: You'll *create* time. And that's all we really want, right? We all desire more time—more time with our loved ones, more time to pursue our passions. But once our time is gone, we can't get it back.

So that's what we aim to do with this book: manufacture time. We want to add time to your life now by giving you the tips that we believe have the biggest, most efficient health impact. We'll seek to add time to your life later, time you would never have had if you hadn't picked up this book. Every minute you invest now pays off with many more to come.

We've tapped into all of our collective knowledge, scoured the medical literature, and talked to some of the top experts in the industry for tips, suggestions, and strategies that have maximum impact in minimum time. We'll teach you how to get the best care possible from your own doctors—how to ask educated questions, get second opinions, be your own best advocate—as well as arm you with the most credible, authoritative, useful, up-to-date information and advice so you can become the healthiest you possible.

All the while, we'll look for the most fun, simplest, and most pleasurable ways to do these things. Because good health doesn't have to mean a bowl of sprouts and 100,000 hours of cardio—it could mean a glass of really fine pinot noir enjoyed under the stars with your partner or best friend. (In fact, research suggests that spending quality time with someone you love might keep you healthier than almost anything else you can do!)

In all of our rushing around, we sometimes neglect the most elemental truth of humanity: We only have one body and one life on this earth. It's up to us to do everything we can to protect it, enjoy it, and make it last as long as we can.

So, are you with us? We're all in this together. When it comes to your best health, let's not waste another minute.

Chapter One

Take 5

In 2005, a very scary article was published in the prestigious medical journal *The New England Journal of Medicine*. Written by 10 of the best-respected researchers in epidemiology—the study of which factors affect the health and illness of entire human populations—the article's title was "A Potential Decline in Life Expectancy in the United States in the 21st Century."

The researchers analyzed data from numerous studies that together involved hundreds of thousands of people and found that, contrary to the upward trend in longevity that has been the norm for centuries, the average person born today might actually die sooner than his or her parents or grandparents did. Despite all the huge advances in medical research and technology—vaccines, antibiotics, organ transplants, mapping the human genome—all of our predicted gains in longevity might be undone by one condition: obesity.

Sure, in the 21st century, we don't have to chop wood for the fire. Or haul water from the well. Or stalk and kill a wild buffalo for meat.

But by sparing ourselves this routine physical labor and feeding ourselves low-quality, easily acquired fast foods, we may have actually time-saved our way into a shorter life here on earth.

From Time-Savers to Time-Creators

The researchers who performed this landmark review cited some other factors that might also trim our country's longevity rate. Sure, a pandemic flu would do the trick. And, of course, pollution could take its toll. Or hospital-acquired antibiotic-resistant pathogens—such as MRSA—could gang up on us and take over.

But not all of the factors they identified were scary apocalyptic outbreaks beyond our individual control. The researchers also cited the significant risks that accompany a lack of regular exercise and ineffective blood pressure screening. They listed tobacco use. Excess stress.

In other words, like obesity, things we can do something about. Things we can take control of. Things we need only become aware of so we can implement changes to make our lives better, healthier, happier, and most likely, longer.

When we look carefully at what this research tells us, it's clear that the solution to turning around this negative trend is not to go back to the Stone Age. The solution is to look at the changes we've made and then reclaim the activities that have the greatest health benefits—doing yard work, tending a kitchen garden, eating home-cooked meals, walking to school or work—while we also take advantage of the brand-new advances in medical science that can make us even healthier.

That's right: We're going to reverse some of those unhealthy time-savers. But we're also going to adopt something new: healthy time-creators.

The Secrets of Vibrant Health

We're so focused on the immediate—Twitter updates, drive-thrus with 60-second guarantees—we can forget each of those individual moments combine to become, hopefully, a very long life. If we take a different perspective on our lives—the long view—

PLAYING THE ODDS   How Many Years?

Every one of our behaviors can be a net positive or negative in terms of our longevity—and the quality of those years. Take a look at the impact of some of the health behaviors at both ends of the health spectrum.

Behavior or condition	How many years?
Smoking	−5 years
High blood pressure	−5 years
Diabetes	−5 years
Obesity	−5 years
Regular exercise	+5 years

we'll see how the choices we make in each of those seconds really do accumulate.

Most of us say we'd make better health choices if we had more time. But perhaps opting for the quick and easy Big Mac or Big Gulp a few too many times in your life has left you with some physical souvenirs—extra pounds, inches, or units of blood sugar. Perhaps skipping routine tests, such as a mammogram, cholesterol test, flu shot, or yearly physical (as the Centers for Disease Control and Prevention says 80 percent of women and 60 percent of men do), may have saved you an hour here or there, but now you're left with an even more serious problem—a lump, the pain of angina, or a dangerous case of pneumonia—to contend with.

But here's the good news: Just as those negative choices can accumulate and snowball into something larger, so can positive ones. And by making one small choice—what we call a health fix—and then another, and then another, your very small choices can add up to big changes.

Live Long and Prosper

We all want to live for a long time—but what fun is it to live a long life if you're stricken with debilitating diseases that cause you pain and suffering?

With this thought in mind, rather than look exclusively for things that prolong life, we also looked at research on what enhances overall health—what makes people healthier and happier, not just live longer.

We looked at dozens of longevity and healthy-aging studies from all over the world. We looked for patterns of behavior and outcomes that transcended all cultures. Luckily, the medical literature abounds with helpful information—most of it underscoring the same points over and over.

One of the most interesting studies helped us by defining this longest, healthiest life as "exceptional aging." The researchers described exceptional aging as living to an advanced age without cognitive or physical impairment or having any of six major chronic diseases—coronary heart disease, stroke, cancer (excluding nonmelanoma skin cancer), chronic obstructive pulmonary disease, Parkinson's disease, and treated diabetes. The researchers chose these six diseases primarily because they are among the most common age-associated chronic conditions. The study, published in *JAMA: The Journal of the American Medical Association,* followed a group of 5,820 men for 40 years. Researchers found one out of every two men who avoided the big-six conditions made it to age 85—but among those who didn't, only one in 10 lived that long.

The exceptional survivors had many things in common. They were more likely than those who'd died earlier to have:

- greater grip strength
- a healthy weight
- lower blood sugar levels
- lower triglyceride levels
- healthy blood pressure
- no history of smoking
- no history of heavy drinking
- a spouse
- more than 12 years of education

This list gave us a great jumping-off point. Considering that many men never make it to age 85—by that age, women outnumber men by 2.2 to 1 in the United States—we agreed that those were findings we should pay attention to.

We looked at many studies just like that one. As we examined their areas of overlap, we zeroed in on 10 key factors that kept rising to the top as the most critical to a long life of health and vitality.

Healthy heart: Since cardiovascular disease is the number one cause of death in America, it stands to reason that the world's healthiest people avoid heart disease—and most do this by adopting lifestyle choices that also benefit the other nine key factors of health.

Healthy brain: Through what scientists believe is a combination of good genes and those same smart lifestyle choices that protect the heart, the world's healthiest people are able to avoid neurological damage, cognitive decline, and Alzheimer's disease.

Healthy lungs: The world's healthiest people safeguard their respiratory health, primarily by avoiding smoking—still the leading *preventable* cause of death in the world—as well as steering clear of environmental and industrial pollution.

Healthy gut and immune system: The healthiest people in all cultures eat fresh, whole foods, mostly vegetables and fruits, and enjoy healthy digestion—which leads to enhanced immunity and lower incidences of cancer.

Healthy bones, muscles, and skin: The world's healthiest people take pains to prevent skin cancer, protect their bones (lessening the likelihood of developing osteoporosis and the debilitating frailty that can spell disaster for older folks), and maintain the muscle mass that allows them to enjoy higher activity levels as they get older (which, in turn, benefits all systems of the body).

Healthy hormones: In seeking balance in their lifestyle—with those smart diet, exercise, and stress management choices that also protect their heart and brain—and by negotiating life's hormonal milestones without extreme interventions, the world's healthiest people maintain a normal hormonal equilibrium, especially avoiding diabetes.

Healthy weight: The world's healthiest people maintain a stable, healthy weight for most of their lives, preventing excessive fluctuations (either gaining or losing)—especially avoiding childhood obesity and staving off weight gain during middle age.

Healthy relationships: Perhaps more importantly than any other factor, the world's healthiest people have loving relationships with their family, friends, and themselves, and they tend to avoid harmful negative emotions such as hostility and hopelessness. Instead they are, by nature or by choice, optimistic people who tend to surround themselves with similarly positive, proactive people.

Healthy pregnancies: The healthiest people on earth are the products of safe, well-cared-for mothers who had access to good nutrition during their relatively stress-free, healthy pregnancies—which, naturally, start with strong sperm and eggs. While we may not be able to turn back the hands of time to affect our own fetal experiences, we can have a huge impact on our children's futures by taking care of our own reproductive health today.

PLAYING THE ODDS

One shocking study, published in the *Archives of Internal Medicine*, looked at 2,357 doctors who were part of the Physicians' Health Study, 970 of whom had lived to age 90. (Naturally, we were especially curious about these findings!) The study concluded that if the doctors had avoided smoking, diabetes, obesity, hypertension, and a sedentary lifestyle by age 70, they had a 54 percent chance of making it to 90.

If they had two of these factors, their odds wavered somewhere between 22 and 36 percent.

If they had five, they basically had no shot—their odds of living to 90 were a nearly nonexistent 4 percent.

Hmmm . . . in one scenario, your odds of living to age 90 are better than one in two. In another scenario, your odds drop to one in 25.

What to do?

We'll tell you what: Start today. Once you've quit smoking (you will, won't you?), you can start addressing the other four factors with one simple remedy: daily exercise.

Healthy childhood: The world's healthiest people are born into conditions that support a healthy childhood, such as access to high-quality food, low levels of environmental toxins, and ample love and support—all of which set them up for a lifetime of good health.

Each of these 10 factors is a powerful health predictor in itself—and when added together, they can improve the quality and extend the length of your life by many years.

How many, you might wonder?

Well, once we had assembled this group of factors, we took a moment to look at studies on twins. We were looking for the differences between genes and environment and how much impact our lifestyle choices make. These studies revealed that our expected life span is likely determined 30 percent by our genes and 70 percent by our lifestyle. And, based on the typical American lifestyle, we're robbing ourselves of an average of *10 years*.

Ten years!

That's a lot of time!

Small Change: It's Worth Collecting

Okay—be honest. Do you think making changes in these 10 areas of health sounds like a lot of work?

We were concerned that you might think that, so we went and found the studies to back up what our 78 years of collective medical experience have shown us. The long-term studies suggest we can make significant gains in our longevity and future vitality by making very small changes.

Here's what you need to know: All the factors we just mentioned can be impacted today, in the next 5 minutes, to change the course of our health both for ourselves and for future generations.

Consider these findings.

Trade one piece of candy for an apple—and save your own life. Researchers found that if every person in the United Kingdom swapped just one single unhealthy snack (such as chips or candy) for a healthy one (such as a piece of fruit) every day, 6,000 deaths from cardiovascular disease could be prevented every year.

Slowing down a mere 1.8 miles per hour can add a week and a half to your life. Yes—driving slower can be a health choice. In a study published in the journal *Medical Decision Making,* scientists found that 1 hour spent behind the wheel of a car was equal to 20 minutes of lost life expectancy due to the potential for a crash—and every 0.6 miles per hour of speed decreases your life expectancy. Why? Any time you save by traveling faster is more than offset by the risk of a crash. Just decreasing your speed by 1.8 miles per hour could save you 3.6 hours each year, which adds up to a week and a half over the average lifetime.

Make nuts your daily snack at work—and live an extra 2 years. A study from Loma Linda University in California of more than 34,000 people found that those who ate nuts five or more times a week lived an extra 1.5 to 2.5 years. Other studies have found that people who eat nuts have 35 to 50 percent lower rates of coronary events such as heart attacks, probably due to nuts' cholesterol-lowering effects and immunity-enhancing antioxidant content.

Trade some chips for an apple. Slow down less than 2 miles per hour. Eat a handful of nuts.

We don't know—does that sound like too much?

If so, let's talk about those 10 years again.

Are you willing to do without them?

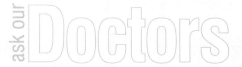

How much more time do I have?

When we speak with our patients about making small steps to gain more years of life, we're often surprised that some folks don't seem to "get" it—they act as if they are the exceptions.

"My mom smoked until she was 85. I'm not going to get lung cancer."

"I hate vegetables. I'd rather die early than eat them."

Really? You'd give up time on earth simply to avoid some broccoli now and then? Well, in that case, take a look at where you stand right now. Try this life expectancy calculator developed by professors from the University of Pennsylvania in Philadelphia and Singapore Management University: http://gosset.wharton.upenn.edu/mortality/perl/CalcForm.html.

You'll learn about some fascinating trade-offs.

For example, if a 50-year-old woman who currently sleeps 6 hours a night bumps that up by just 1 extra hour, she will gain almost 7 extra months of life. If that same woman currently has two or three drinks a day and cuts down to one, she'll gain 7 months and 11 days. And if she's a couch potato, adopting a rigorous "conditioning" exercise program will give her the biggest gain—she could live an extra 2 years, 8 months, and 2 weeks.

Try it and see—your gains for making small changes might be even more dramatic. Not a bad trade for time-creators that also give you more strength, energy, and vitality during those extra years.

Or do you think a few minutes here and there might be a good trade-off to gain extra years of life on the back end?

We do. And we think you agree. That's why we're here to make these 5-minute fixes as easy, pleasurable, and fun as we possibly can.

How to Use This Book

We know that in our daily lives, the long term can seem a long way off. And between shuttling the kids to soccer practice and racing to make deadlines at work, safeguarding your health can become an afterthought, just another thing on an endless to-do list. But health doesn't need to be hard, or take a lot of time.

Now, in case you've already taken a sneak peek at some of the following chapters, we want to reassure you—we're not suggesting that you have to do all of these fixes. We're not even suggesting that you do most of them. If you only do one, that's a start! We know from our experience with thousands of patients that as soon you make one healthy change, you're more likely to add others.

This fact was heavily underscored by our research as well: We saw, in study after study, that people who engaged in one healthy behavior were more likely to engage in two. Those who engaged in two were more likely to engage in three. And so on, on and on.

That's how health is—it's cumulative. You make a change, you stick with that change, and the effects pile up. You make another change, and that effect also accumulates. Start where you are, change one thing today, and then keep going. With each 5-minute fix you do, you're adding hours and days and years to the back end.

As you make your way through the book, you can either read from one chapter to the next, collecting information and insight as you go, or you can simply open it up to any chapter that appeals to you and start there. All the systems in the body are interconnected, so making a change for the better in any key area will have a positive ripple effect throughout your body—and your life. Make enough ripples and you'll soon be riding a wave of good health!

On Your Marks, Get Ready . . .

Before you begin, we want to caution you: You may be tempted to jump in and do a bunch of things all at once. And that's okay—exuberance and enthusiasm, especially when it comes to health and self-care, can be tremendously motivating! But for those who prefer a slower, more gradual approach, or for those who may have started other "plans" with a bang but are now a bit burned out, we suggest taking a kinder, gentler path to health.

ask our **Doctors**

I want to make sure I get the most out of my doctor's visits, but I always leave without feeling like my questions have been answered. What should I do?

Dr. Travis says . . .

I love this question—I wish every patient would learn how to take full advantage of physical examinations.

First, I suggest that you write everything down before you go. Being nervous for a doctor's visit is completely normal and it can make you forget important things to discuss. Speak up during your appointment and write down things you don't want to forget (especially information about follow-up treatment, like when to take your medications and any side effects you should expect).

Your physician isn't a mind reader, and if you have concerns you need to express them. He or she won't judge your health history regardless of how you may feel about it. Being honest will help your physician properly diagnose you.

Finally, don't be afraid to call back after you leave. If you forget to ask a question, it's okay to leave a voice mail message for (or send an e-mail to) your doctor or nurse-practitioner. The most important thing is that you have a good, open, trusting relationship with your doctor and the other staff members in his or her practice.

While we were writing this book, we were continually reminded of the philosophy of Kaizen. Originally a Japanese business philosophy, Kaizen—which translates as "improvement" or "change for the better"—focuses on the idea that small steps toward quality, when taken continuously, will add up to big results. The idea is not that everything should be scrapped so a whole new company (or, in your case, a whole new life) can be started, but rather that the most effective means of change is to start right where you are and to fine-tune—to optimize your current system.

This Eastern philosophy dovetails perfectly with countless Western scientific studies that have shown that behavioral changes that are made incrementally last longer. And that's what you want—permanent changes that will help you feel stronger, more vibrant, more alive; that leave you with more energy and enthusiasm; that let you get more pleasure out of every part of your life.

Doctors' orders: It's time to take 5—and recharge your life.

Chapter Two
Have a Heart

Lub-dub. Lub-dub. Lub-dub. We fell in love with that sound in the womb, when Mom's heartbeat was the soundtrack of our lives for 9 months. And no matter our age, that sound—the steady, rhythmic sound of the heartbeat—is one of the most soothing on earth.

As we go through our day, we're often not even conscious of it. When we do take a second to key in to that rhythm, it can seem as steady and simple as a ticking clock. But what's happening behind that sound is one of the most complex and critical biological processes in our bodies.

A 5-Minute Tour of Your Heart

The heart is, by definition, our most important organ—when it conks out, it's game over. Where the heart goes, so goes our health. When we're looking for small changes that might have big results in the rest of our lives, we'll start right here.

A healthy heart is the general of a healthy, thriving cardiovascular system, a well-oiled machine composed of two parts:

- The heart (the "cardio"), a pump that acts on the bidding of the brain, responding to electrical signals to keep your blood moving in the right direction—oxygen-rich blood out to all frontiers of the body and oxygen-depleted blood back to the lungs to be recharged and sent back out again
- The blood vessels (the "vascular"), the tubes that carry this blood everywhere from your pinkie toes to your cerebral cortex

The heart is ambidextrous—the right and left sides work at exactly the same time but with different functions, to distribute blood to the body. In order for this process to work as it should, our 16,000 miles of blood vessels have to remain limber and clear so the blood flows through them easily. And each of the valves between the four chambers of the heart have to open and close at exactly the right times to send the blood along its appointed path.

That's a lot to ask of such a small organ! But we often expect our hearts to function like stalwart postal workers on their routes—neither stress, nor smoke, nor greasy foods should stop them from doing their critical work. The sad truth is, one day, your own little stalwart postal worker will grow weary—and if you don't take good care of it now, that postal worker could be headed for an early retirement.

Fix It in 5
Reduce Your Risk of Heart Disease

1. Commit yourself to heart-healthy nutrition.
2. Enjoy physical activity daily.
3. Stop using tobacco in any form and avoid secondhand smoke.
4. Control diabetes by closely monitoring blood sugar and losing excess weight.
5. Stick with the heart-healthy plan you and your doctor devise and keep him or her well informed of any changes in your health if you have a family history of heart disease.

Keep the Pipes Clear

Imagine a pipe at the kitchen faucet: The flow of water slows and then stops, and you have no water for the important task you were going to do. Clogged arteries can cause similar problems, and sometimes result in a complete stoppage. When a block like this is in the heart, it starves the heart tissue of oxygen, causing a heart attack. (When a similar stoppage happens in the brain, you have a stroke.)

What's a major cause of those clogged arterial pipes? Inflammation.

Recent research demonstrates that inflammation is the mechanism that causes the blockage to start, grow, and finally block the blood vessel entirely. Throughout this book, you will learn the things you can do to decrease inflammation: quit smoking, lower your blood sugar, lower your blood pressure, lose weight, exercise, reduce stress, and love life! And, equally important, lower your cholesterol.

Now, hang on. Before you go swearing off egg yolks, you should know that, while dietary cholesterol has a bad reputation, our bodies actually need it to make hormones and cell membranes. Only about one-quarter of the cholesterol in our bodies comes from our food—the rest is manufactured by the liver and other cells. The problems start when excess cholesterol starts roaming through our arteries and getting stuck in the walls. As that buildup (called plaque) increases, it can block the artery, making it stiff and impassable—and lead to the kind of trouble that can shorten by years, even decades, those long lives we seek.

When you get a blood test to check your cholesterol level, you used to be given one number—your total cholesterol—which, hopefully, was under 200. But although we once simply looked at the total cholesterol level, now we know that all cholesterol is not created equal.

Low-density lipoprotein, also known as LDL, is the "bad" kind. LDL molecules combine with other substances to form a thick, hard plaque on the insides of your arteries, a condition called atherosclerosis. When it builds up enough, that deposit forms a clot—the clog in the drain—that can back up the blood flow and starve your heart or brain of critical oxygen.

High-density lipoprotein, also known as HDL, is the "good" kind. These molecules haul away cholesterol and bring it to the liver to be removed from the body. HDL may even grab extra cholesterol from the arterial walls, skimming away some of that dangerous plaque buildup. The higher your HDL level, the better—for every 5 points your HDL rises, your heart disease risk drops by 25 percent.

Triglycerides are similar to LDL in that they can gunk up arteries if there are too many floating around in the bloodstream. Triglycerides are energy boosters—when the body consumes calories, it stores the leftovers that aren't immediately used by the body for use later on, and that package of energy is called a triglyceride. This mechanism can be quite useful for marathon runners, for example, who need a continuous source of energy and don't have the ability to eat more food during races. But those of us who eat lunch and then sit around for the rest of the day probably never use those energy boosters, so they end up floating around, unneeded, in our bloodstream, mucking up the works.

Keep the Pump Working

In addition to keeping the vessels clear, your pump needs to remain powerful enough to move blood through your body 24 hours a day, 7 days a week, without ever taking a break. By not doing any exercise, a couch potato is training his or her heart to be weak and unable to pump vigorously. But the good news is, once you start exercising, your muscles gain strength, and the muscle that makes up your heart does too. Anything that makes your heart pump harder—walking, climbing stairs, crazy dancing with your kids—will help keep it strong and capable of handling its 24/7 pumping job.

When a heart is pumping properly, it creates a lot of force that pushes blood through your blood vessels. The force of that pressure is called systole, and it creates the *ba-bump* you feel under your fingertips when you take your pulse—this is the first, "systolic" part of your blood pressure reading. The pressure in your arteries during the downtime between beats, when the heart is relaxed, is called the diastolic pressure. When the heart is actively pumping, the pressure is higher, which is why the systolic number is higher than the diastolic.

Now, while dietary cholesterol may not be as fearsome a foe as was once suspected, salt is actually starting to look worse and worse—especially the excessive added salt in processed foods. Why is it bad? Eating excess salt causes fluid retention, which means your heart has more blood to pump through the same small blood vessels (capillaries). This increases pressure and places extra stress on your heart and blood vessels.

Unfortunately, we might never know we have high blood pressure (also called hypertension). Because it has so few symptoms, high blood pressure is called the silent killer. Uncontrolled high blood pressure can lead to heart problems, such as heart attacks or heart failure, but it can also lead to stroke or kidney failure. According to the University of Maryland Medical Center in Baltimore, half of Americans have high blood pressure, but only half of them know it. And of that half, only half are controlling it well. Do the math: That means three out of four people with high blood pressure are at high risk for dangerous outcomes. Are you one of them?

Some of the factors we cannot control include a family history of hypertension, our age (being over 55 as a female or 44 as a male), existing kidney disease, or African American heritage. But other than that, there are lots of factors we can control, either in part or completely.

FACTORS WE CAN PARTIALLY CONTROL

- Are you around people who smoke every day? (You could work with them on a smoking cessation program, in part by telling them how dangerous their smoking is for you.)
- Are you diabetic or prediabetic? Is your fasting glucose more than 100 mg/dL? (You could work with your doctor on developing a diet and exercise program that will help you get better control of your blood sugar.)
- Do you have high cholesterol? (You could work with your doctor on a diet and exercise program that will help you decrease LDL and increase HDL cholesterol.)

FACTORS WE CAN CONTROL

- Are you a smoker? (You can quit with the help of your doctor, local or online smoking cessation groups, a firm commitment to your health, and perhaps even nicotine patches or gum.)
- Are you overweight or obese? (You can eat more nutritious, whole foods and exercise more often.)
- Are you sedentary? (You can move your body at least 30 minutes most days of the week.)
- Are you taking oral contraceptives? (You can talk to your doctor about alternative contraceptive methods.)
- Are you a woman who has more than one drink a day? (You can cut down, either by yourself or with the help of your doctor or other support group.)
- Are you a man who has more than two drinks a day? (You can cut down, either by yourself or with the help of your doctor or other support group.)

All of us should have our blood pressure checked every time we see our physicians. But if you answered yes to several of these questions, consider buying your own blood pressure monitor. You can get an inexpensive one for as little as $10 at a discount store. Track your blood pressure and watch for patterns—does it jump up during March Madness? Does it head downward during your vacation?

Don't be alarmed if your blood pressure fluctuates over the course of the day—that's entirely normal and may be quite healthy. You're simply collecting information. Track it in a small notebook or use an online tracker such as the one available at the American Heart Association's www.heart360.org. Taking your own blood pressure is an excellent way to get in tune with your heart—and your whole body.

Keep Inflammation Down

We all know that eating fatty foods can clog arteries, but the fat in the food does not literally travel from the food into your blood vessels. So the question is, what is the connection? Enter inflammation, another known risk factor for clogged arteries. Inflammation is triggered when our body takes certain cues from our environment (like smoking, elevated blood sugar, excess weight, stress, and others) and reacts with the inflammatory response. The body starts sending in reinforcements with the best of intentions—to first stop harm being done by negative forces that cued the response and then to begin the process of healing. Inflammation, then, may be one of the root causes of atherosclerosis, the buildup of plaque in the arteries.

When blood vessels are damaged by any of the events mentioned above, the body may be reacting in the same way as when you cut your finger or contract a virus. Doctors can detect inflammation in blood vessels by measuring C-reactive protein, or CRP, a protein whose production increases during systemic inflammation. When your body has high levels of CRP, it's a sign that damage has occurred in your vessels that might lead to clogged arteries and heart attacks or strokes.

TESTING YOUR BLOOD PRESSURE

If you're under a cardiologist's care, he or she might ask you to get an at-home blood pressure monitor to keep track of your stats and stay on top of any incremental rises. Bring your monitor to your next doctor's visit, and ask the nurse to teach you how to use it and to make sure it's accurate. Make sure you:

- Avoid food, caffeine, alcohol, exercise, and tobacco for at least 30 minutes before the test
- Use the bathroom first
- Roll up your sleeve and securely wrap the cuff around your biceps, a little above your elbow and on the bare skin
- Sit calmly and quietly in a comfortable seat with a back, with your arm elevated near heart level (not hanging down). Keep your feet flat on the floor and breathe deeply.

The top, higher number—the systolic blood pressure reading—is the maximum pressure generated as the heart beats or contracts. The bottom, lower number—the diastolic blood pressure reading—is the pressure in the arteries when the heart rests between beats.

SYSTOLIC PRESSURE (TOP NUMBER)	DIASTOLIC PRESSURE (BOTTOM NUMBER)	HEALTH STATUS	ACTIONS NEEDED
Consistently below 90	Consistently below 60	Possibly hypotensive	Check with your doctor—healthy young women may have BP below 90/60, but others may have an underlying medical condition
90–115	60–75	Perfect!	Keep doing what you're doing!
116–119	76–79	Normal	Okay for now—but stay vigilant with heart-health fixes
120–139	80–89	Prehypertensive	At your next physical, ask your doctor about steps you can take to head off any major concerns
140–159	90–99	High blood pressure, stage 1	Talk to your doctor within the next week
160 or higher	100 or higher	High blood pressure, stage 2	Call your doctor today

WARNING SIGN! HEART ATTACK

"Am I having a heart attack?" is one of the most common questions that brings people to the ER. And while many people feel embarrassed when their symptoms turn out to be false alarms, we always reassure people—better safe than sorry. And the faster the better. During the first hour of a heart attack, you are most at risk for sudden death and your heart sustains the most damage. But if you're treated quickly, you'll have the most options for dealing with the crisis and be in the best position to make a full recovery.

Heart attacks can be triggered by stress, a very high-fat meal, sporadic vigorous activity (such as shoveling snow after sitting on your butt for 4 months), even the time of day—heart attacks occur more often between 4 a.m. and 10 a.m. than any other six-hour period.

Some of the most common symptoms of heart attack include:

- an uncomfortable pressure or sensation of squeezing, fullness, or pain in the center of the chest that lasts for more than a few minutes or goes away and comes back
- discomfort in other areas of the upper body, such as one or both of the arms, the back, the neck, the jaw, or the abdomen
- shortness of breath, which often occurs with or before chest discomfort
- heartbeat sensations that feel like your heart is pounding or racing
- a cold sweat
- nausea or vomiting
- light-headedness or fainting
- anxiety or a sense of impending doom

Some people—especially older folks, those with diabetes, and women—can have additional or slightly different symptoms with a heart attack.

- abdominal pain
- unusual or unexplained fatigue
- little or no chest pain

Heart attacks can masquerade as a multitude of different ailments, and vice versa. True, you may be having a panic attack or a fainting episode. You may even have simple indigestion. If you're concerned, please call 911 and follow the directions of the operator. You'll soon be in good hands.

5 Minute Fixes
for a Lifetime of Heart Health

Maintaining a healthy amount of pressure in your blood vessels, keeping them clear of obstructions, and making sure you have a strong pump are the keys to good cardiovascular health. The World Health Organization estimates that we lose 2,115 years of healthy life each year in the United States due to cardiovascular diseases. While some problems with heart health do run in families, most do not: Research has shown that as many as 80 percent of heart attacks are preventable. If you're looking for a focus for your healthy-living efforts, you can't ask for a better target than your heart. Heart-healthy habits automatically lower your risks of many other dangerous chronic diseases, such as diabetes, cancer, and Alzheimer's.

That's why the tips below are the ultimate time-savers: Every single one of these heart-health fixes can cause a cascade of positive effects on other aspects of your health. Let's look at some ways you can keep your heart (and the rest of your body) healthy for good.

Book your vacation. Now here's a health fix we can all agree upon! Unfortunately, when economic times are tough, a lot of people skip vacations. But people with a higher risk of heart disease who take a vacation every year are 32 percent less likely to die from heart disease at any time and 30 percent less likely to die of a heart attack specifically. Worried about the money? Consider it a health investment: Research shows you'll be much happier spending it on a vacation than on any "thing" like a television or a new stereo system. Spending money on "stuff" feels good at first, but the buzz wanes quickly. In contrast, when you spend your money on an experience like a vacation or a massage, you feel more positive emotions—which prolong the heart-healthy effect. **Time spent:** 5 minutes to enter dates and credit card info online or book through a travel agent

Now research the destination. Continue to plan your trip for a few minutes a day and you'll increase the heart-healthiness of the trip even before you leave! One Dutch study found that up to 16 weeks before a planned vacation, the anticipation of the big trip can increase feelings of happiness—which, with its ability to reduce belly-fat-creating stress hormones such as cortisol, is always good for your heart. (This anticipation can actually make you even happier than you'll be during the trip itself.) **Time spent:** 5 fun minutes a day

Schedule a blood test. Denial is the enemy of good heart health. The first step to understanding is to know your current health status—and that starts with a blood test. When you phone your doctor's office to schedule your annual checkup (you're doing that, right?), save time by asking them to mail or fax you a prescription for a blood test called a blood lipid profile, so you can get it done before your office visit. (Check out the recommended tests listed at the back of the book to set your targets.) **Time spent:** 1 minute to request the prescription and 4 minutes to schedule the blood test

Smear ½ teaspoon of butter on your white bread treat. New research from Italy suggests that we should pay attention to the speed of our carbohydrates: In a study including more than 32,000 women, those whose diets had the highest glycemic load—the measure of how quickly a food elevates the blood sugar level—had more than twice the risk of heart disease as those whose diets had the lowest glycemic load. Eating a diet with more healthful, complex carbohydrates—love those veggies, fruits, and whole grains!—helps women reduce their risk of heart disease in part by avoiding the high triglycerides and lowered HDL levels that are more significant risk factors for women than men.

Sometimes the trick to lowering your glycemic load is to strategically add a bit more food. By ensuring that your meal includes a bit of protein or fiber (or even a nutrient heart patients have traditionally been scolded to avoid, fat), you can slow down your body's insulin release, keeping your blood sugar stable. For example, if you're having grapes for a snack, you could eat a cheese stick at the same time. Smear your PB&J bread with more protein-packed peanut butter, less sugar-filled jelly. If you really want to treat yourself to a piece of white bread at dinner, smear it with (gasp!) half a pat of butter—that lowers the bread's glycemic index of 72 to 59. (Just don't do it very often!)

To lower the overall average glycemic load of your diet, as often as possible, reach for foods waaaay down on the glycemic index: Lentils, lean chicken, fish, fresh greens, broccoli, cabbage, walnuts. Choose cherries over cantaloupe, an apple over pineapple. Then, when you have that fresh bread treat, it won't throw you off by much. **Time spent:** 20 decadent seconds

Lie in bed an extra minute. And take your resting heart rate. Your pulse—the rate at which your heart pumps blood through your arteries—can tell you a lot about your overall health, and your resting heart rate, when taken upon awakening in the morning, is a great indicator of cardiac fitness. As a person's cardiovascular health improves, his or her resting pulse tends to decrease. To find your resting heart rate:

- Put a watch or clock with a second hand on your bedside table before you go to sleep
- Allow your body to wake up gently the next morning (i.e., not with an alarm clock!)
- Place your index and middle fingers on the inner side of your wrist, toward your thumb
- Feel for a pulsing sensation under your fingers
- When you find it, look at the clock and wait until the second hand hits the 12
- Count your pulse until the second hand hits the 6
- Double that number; that's your heart rate

Most adults' resting heart rates fall in the 60 to 80 beats per minute (bpm) range, but your risk of heart attack is greatly increased when your resting heart rate is 70 or above. One study found that subjects' odds of developing a diabetes-related illness rose 10 percent for each extra 12 bpm when compared with those who had the lowest heart rates. **Time spent:** 30 seconds to take your pulse, 30 seconds to calculate your bpm

Double the distance. Starting today, you're going to put away that pointing finger—you know, the one that presses the button for the elevator—and take the stairs. In an office building, trading the elevator for the stairs is a no-brainer. But even if you only have one flight of stairs in your house, you can double its power: Every time you go up or down, automatically turn around and double it. Do that 20 times a day and you've climbed 300 extra stairs, which equates to 5 extra minutes of activity and 50 extra calories burned each day. (Boom—that's 5 pounds gone this year.) **Time spent:** 15 seconds each time, 20 times a day = 5 minutes

Reset your default calendar reminder. If you have an electronic calendar that "pings" you 5 minutes before meetings, set it to give you 5 minutes longer than that—and then use that time to take an extra turn around the hallway, parking lot, or block before the meeting. Just scroll to your calendar software's Preferences to set up your "fitness fix" reminder. **Time spent:** 1 minute to change the reminder, 5 minutes for walking

Pour yourself a cup—or four. A recent long-term study of 130,000 men and women 18 to 90 years old found that those who drank 4 or more cups of coffee a day had an almost 18 percent lower risk of heart rhythm disturbances. Think 4 cups sounds like a recipe for the jitters? That "dosage" of coffee may yield the greatest benefits to your heart. A National Institutes of Health (NIH) study of more than 86,000 women found that those who drank 4 or 5 cups of coffee a day were 26 percent less likely to die from any causes than those who didn't drink coffee at all. (Those who drank just 5 to 7 cups a week had only a 7 percent advantage over nondrinkers.) The kicker? The java fiends' longer lives may be mostly thanks to their reduced risk of cardiovascular disease. Check with your doctor—and, once you get his or her okay, enjoy that coffee guilt-free! **Time spent:** 2 minutes to pour an extra cup or two

But put away the French press first. As the good news about drinking coffee piles up—it decreases risks of type 2 diabetes, liver problems, Parkinson's disease, some forms of cancer—

we are learning that the type of coffee you drink matters. An organic compound called cafestol that is found in unfiltered coffee can dramatically raise your level of LDL, the "bad" cholesterol. Research suggests that if you drink 5 cups of French press coffee per day for 4 weeks, you could raise your cholesterol by up to 8 percent. The filter in drip coffeemakers removes most of the cafestol—and, bonus, drip makers take less time to brew than French presses do.

(Note that reusable gold filters don't catch cafestol, so to maximize the heart-healthy benefits of coffee, and minimize any potential risks, replace your gold filter with unbleached paper filters. Faster cleanup, and better for your heart!) **Time spent:** 2 minutes to stash your French press and get out the drip machine and paper filters

Buy a split instead of a regular-size bottle of wine. These single-serve wine bottles are the perfect way to drink the right portion for your heart. According to Mehdi Razavi, MD, cardiologist with the Texas Heart Institute in Houston, every ounce of alcohol you drink increases your blood pressure by 10 points and increases your risk of irregular heartbeats. When it comes to alcohol, red wine is certainly always your best choice—studies have suggested that antioxidants in red wine called polyphenols help protect the lining of blood vessels in your heart. But there is a limit: More than two 4-ounce glasses of red wine per day for men and one glass per day for women will actually do more harm than good. **Time spent:** zero seconds (it takes the same amount of time to buy any size bottle of wine!)

Don't go crazy with the cocktail math. The cutoff amounts for beer and hard liquor are even lower than for wine—if you are at risk for heart disease (and really, who isn't?), stick to one glass of wine, beer, or hard liquor per day. And even if you are drinking red wine, you are not allowed to multiply 4 ounces by seven nights in order to justify consuming 14 ounces on Friday and Saturday nights instead of having a glass of wine with dinner during the rest of the week. Occasional heavy drinkers—those who have five or more drinks at least once a month— are actually 45 percent more likely to develop heart disease than those who average a drink or

One

Supplement, 14 Benefits
Fish Oil

Probably the most compelling indication of fish oil's power is the fact that many doctors take it themselves: A Wake Forest University study found that after attending a course on herbs and dietary supplements, doctors increased their personal usage of fish oil by 30 percent—more than any other supplement (some of which they actually lessened their use of).

Evidence continues to pile up that increasing our intake of omega-3s, the essential fatty acids in fish oil, can help us prevent or reverse some of the most dangerous chronic diseases—and even aging itself. A recent study from the University of California at San Francisco of more than 600 people with heart disease found that those with high levels of omega-3s in their blood appeared to be younger on a chromosomal level than those with lower levels of them. Their telomeres—the ends of chromosomes that help the body repair cellular damage—were longer, making them better able to keep tissues healthy. Other benefits linked to high omega-3 levels include:

1. Lower blood pressure in hypertensive people
2. Raised HDL ("good") cholesterol level
3. Reduced risk of death, heart attack, dangerous abnormal heart rhythms, and strokes in people who've had a heart attack
4. Slowed hardening of the arteries
5. Decreased inflammation
6. Slower genetic aging, specifically in heart patients
7. Reduced joint pain in people with rheumatoid arthritis
8. Improved kidney function
9. Reduced macular degeneration
10. Decreased risk of developing breast, colon, or prostate cancer
11. When used in conjunction with other treatment, relief of some symptoms of postpartum depression, childhood depression, schizophrenia, and bipolar disorder
12. Decreased risk of cognitive decline
13. Enhanced infant eye and brain development
14. Relief from painful menstruation

The American Heart Association recommends taking at least 1 gram per day of fish oil's eicosapentaenoic acid (EPA) and docosahexaenoic acid (DHA), or 2 to 4 grams of each per day if you have high cholesterol. Ask your doctor what the best dosage is for you. (If you are on any other heart medications or have a blood-clotting disorder, fish oil might cause serious side effects such as uncontrolled bleeding.)

Concerned about heavy metal toxicity due to the high levels of some pollutants in fish? The Environmental Defense Fund did a study of 75 brands of fish oil supplements and found 80 percent of the brands they tested to be safe. The most expensive ones weren't necessarily the best—many generic brands passed with flying colors. Here's a sampling of the safest store brands available (see the full list at www.edf.org):

STORE	PRODUCT/BRAND
A&P	Health Pride
Albertsons	Nature's Valley, Sav-On/Albertsons
Costco	Kirkland
CVS	CVS Pharmacy
Duane Reade	Cod Liver Oil, EPA, Fish Oil
Eckerd	Eckerd
Giant Eagle	Cod Liver Oil, Fish Oil
GNC	Cod Liver Oil, DHA 250, Omega Complex
Kroger/Ralphs	Kroger
Longs	Fish Oil Concentrate
Price Chopper	Cod Liver Oil, Fish Oil
Puritan's Pride	Cod Liver Oil, DHA, EPA, Fish Oil, Halibut Liver Oil, Heart Assure, Joint Maintenance, Omega-3, Shark Liver Oil, Triple Omega
Rexall Sundown	EPA/DHA, Fish Oil, Essential Oils/EFA
Safeway	Safeway Select
Sam's Club	Member's Mark
Shoprite	Cod Liver Oil, Fish Oil
Target	Cod Liver Oil, EPA, Fish Oil, Omega-3
Wegmans	Wegmans

two a day. When it comes to your heart, four times seven does not equal 14 times two. **Time spent**: at least a few minutes a day of extra drinking time

Move the saltshaker to the cupboard. Seventy-five percent of the sodium we consume comes from processed foods and medications—some antacids may contain 5 mg of sodium per tablet! If we then sprinkle more salt over our dinner plates, it's no surprise that we end up ingesting an average 3,436 mg of sodium each day, more than double the recommended cap of 1,500 mg. An easy first step is to eliminate "autopilot" salting: Simply put the saltshaker out of sight. If we could reduce our sodium intake to 2,300 mg per day (which is still pretty high), America could eliminate 11 million cases of hypertension (and save $18 billion on health care!). **Time spent:** 30 seconds to stash the shaker

Crunch up Fiber One for bread crumbs. We learned this trick from Hungry Girl Lisa Lillien when she came on the show: Instead of using traditional bread crumbs to coat baked chicken breasts, chop up General Mills's original Fiber One cereal for a low-calorie, nutrition-packed, crunchy coating. A meta-analysis published in the *American Journal of Clinical Nutrition* found that every extra gram of soluble fiber in your daily diet—and a ½-cup serving of Fiber One has 1 gram of soluble fiber—can trim your LDL cholesterol by almost 2 mg/dL. Other sources of soluble fiber include oat bran, oatmeal, beans, peas, barley, citrus fruits, pears, and apple pulp. **Time spent:** 3 minutes to crush cereal into crumbs

Swap fat-free Greek yogurt for sour cream. The DASH diet—a landmark eating plan of "Dietary Approaches to Stop Hypertension" developed by the NIH—includes plenty of calcium, a mineral that helps maintain healthy blood pressure. Just don't count on sour cream as a source of that calcium—if you typically use 2 tablespoons of sour cream on your burrito or baked potato, you're getting zero calcium and just 2 scant grams of muscle-building protein with those 120 calories and 10 grams of artery-clogging saturated fat. In contrast, tangy, fat-free Greek yogurt has a similar flavor and texture, but it packs almost

15 percent of your daily requirement of calcium and 5 grams of protein into 30 calories—with zero saturated fat. You can use the yogurt in place of sour cream in dips, sauces, and salad dressings—you'll never know the difference. **Time spent:** 1 minute to find the Greek yogurt in the store

Give your main squeeze (at least) two hugs a day. Once we've been with someone for a while, we tend to drop the hug habit when time is tight. But your heart needs that close touch, and it doesn't even have to take that long! Doctors from the University of North Carolina at Chapel Hill found that when happily married women hugged their spouses for 20 seconds, their blood pressure and stress hormone levels dropped and their level of oxytocin—the heart-healthy "cuddle hormone"—increased. We'd imagine you can get this effect from a snug with a very close relative or friend, anyone who supports you and makes you feel loved. **Time spent:** 40 seconds (although we'd prefer much more!)

Have a quickie. Now, we're not going to tell you how long this particular "fix" should last—that's up to you and your partner!—but we can tell you that a man's ability to get an erection is directly related to his arterial health. If you're not able to have that quickie without the help of Viagra (sildenafil) or Cialis (tadalafil), it's time to call a cardiologist. Up to 70 percent of men with cardiovascular disease suffer from erectile dysfunction (ED), versus 20 to 30 percent in the general population. And an international study of more than 1,500 men with heart disease found that those who suffered from ED were twice as likely to have a heart attack as those who did not. Researchers say ED can be a great indicator of underlying cardiovascular disease, but they fear that some guys go to the doctor for Viagra or Cialis and then never see a cardiologist—and while those drugs do increase blood flow, they don't treat the hardening of the arteries that's likely the source of the problem itself. Make time with your honey—or, if you can't, make that call to the cardiologist. **Time spent:** As much as desired (for the quickie) or 2 minutes (for that call to the cardiologist)

ask our Doctors

I know I should quit smoking so I don't get lung cancer. But are smokes really that bad for my heart? Can't I just cut down?

There is no room for equivocation: Avoiding cigarettes means smoking none. Smoking even a single cigarette can initiate a cascade of events that can increase the risk of blood-clot formation in vessels that feed the heart and thereby cause a heart attack. Your goal has to be complete cessation. There are many medications that can aid in this task. Still, I have yet to meet a patient who has been successful without the most important ingredients: determination and self-control. If your spouse smokes, then consider quitting together. It will not be easy, but it will be worth it: One year after your last cigarette, your risk of cardiovascular disease will be the same as a lifelong nonsmoker.

—***Mehdi Razavi, MD,*** *cardiologist at the Texas Heart Institute in Houston*

Take the batteries out of your remote. One Australian study published in *Circulation,* a journal of the American Heart Association, found that every hour of television that you watch each day increases your risk of dying from cardiovascular disease by 18 percent. Every hour! If you watch for 4 hours a day, you increase your risk of premature death by 46 percent. If removing the batteries doesn't cut your TV addiction, try unplugging the set, throwing a tablecloth over it, moving the comfortable furniture away from it—anything to make it less accessible or appealing. If you must watch, set a kitchen timer for 1 hour and then walk or run on a treadmill, do jumping jacks, or even walk in place while watching. Anything to keep yourself up and moving while your mind zones out. **Time spent:** 1 minute to take those batteries out of the remote

Skip the grapefruit—just hit the grape. Grapefruit, apples, and oranges and their juices can prevent our bodies from correctly absorbing medications for cholesterol, blood pressure, and ED. Chemicals in these citrus fruits can interfere with the enzymes necessary to metabolize these drugs. If you're on any of these medications, reach for Concord grape juice instead— research suggests that these dark purple grapes can reduce the risk of blood clots, lower LDL, prevent damage to blood vessels in the heart, and help maintain healthy blood pressure. They also have flavonoids, cancer-fighting antioxidants that may increase HDL, the beneficial cholesterol, and help reduce the risk of clogged arteries. Just be sure to stick with a half-cup serving and dilute grape juice with water or seltzer, because the high sugar content and extra calories could negate any benefit by adding to your visceral fat. **Time spent:** 10 seconds to reach past the grapefruit to select the Concord grape juice instead

Make a happy list. When we get really overwhelmed by how hard life is—the bills! global warming! wars! taxes!—that's when it's even more important to remind ourselves to think positively. That's not just being Pollyannaish—recent research funded by the NIH found that happier people are significantly less likely to develop heart problems. Researchers followed more than 1,700 men and women for 10 years and rated their happiness levels on a 5-point scale. They found that every extra point of happiness corresponded with a 22 percent lower chance of heart problems.

Do this: Turn a piece of paper sideways and, across the top, write five things in your life that make you happy—your dog, your kids, your favorite football team, and so on. Then, under each one, brainstorm all the ways you can increase your enjoyment of those things in 5-minute blocks. (Example: Brush the dog. Play fetch. E-mail my son. Put his picture in a frame. Research the upcoming season. Order a new jersey.) Keep that list nearby for a fast happiness infusion after a hard day. **Time spent:** 5 minutes to write the list today, then 5 more minutes of happiness every day

Sign up for CPR and AED training. If someone you love has significant heart issues, you may find comfort in knowing exactly what to do in an emergency. In the case of cardiac arrest, the chance of survival decreases by 10 percent for every minute without intervention, but if someone administers CPR and AED, odds of survival double or even triple. CPR and AED training is offered by almost every hospital in the country. Check out the American Heart Association's Emergency Cardiovascular Care (ECC) Class Connector at www.americanheart.org to find CPR and AED classes near you. **Time spent:** 5 minutes signing up today (plus several hours of training)

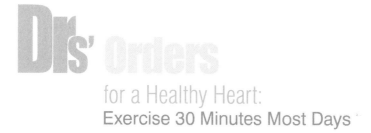

Drs' Orders
for a Healthy Heart:
Exercise 30 Minutes Most Days

Exercise is essential not only to a healthy heart, but also to your future as a human being. Exercise gives you more energy to play with your kids or grandkids; it helps you feel strong and confident enough to dance at a wedding, play volleyball at a picnic, or simply hurry to catch a bus. Couch potatoes are more likely to have arteries that are clogged up with bad cholesterol,

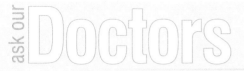
Heart attack, cardiac arrest—what's the difference?

Dr. Travis says . . .

People often use the terms "heart attack" and "cardiac arrest" interchangeably, but they are two very different crises. Cardiac arrest is caused by an abnormal rhythm—an arrhythmia—in the heart's electrical system that causes the heart to suddenly stop. Cardiac arrest (or sudden cardiac death, SCD) strikes in an instant, often without warning.

During cardiac arrest, a person suddenly passes out, does not respond when touched, and does not appear to be breathing. In these situations, call 911, use an AED—an automated external defibrillator—if one is available, and start CPR. AED machines check for a heart rhythm, recognize a rhythm that needs a shock, and guide the rescuer in what steps to take next.

If your workplace does not have an AED—or you have a person with significant heart issues in your home—consider purchasing one. (Visit www.americanheart.org for a list of AED vendors approved by the FDA.)

calcium, and fatty deposits—but exercise lowers your blood pressure, strengthens your heart, helps you manage stress better, and improves your body's ability to use oxygen—which keeps your skin looking rosy, healthy, and supple. Exercise increases your HDL, your body's "good" cholesterol that whisks away artery-clogging gunk and offsets other cardiac risks. Exercise improves your body's ability to move sugar from your blood into your muscles (rather than your fat), helping to prevent diabetes while increasing your calorie-burning muscle mass.

In short, exercise is cardiac medicine—the most effective, efficient, safe, healthy medicine we have—and taking this medicine will determine how many more high-quality years your heart has on this planet.

Your doctor understands that the daily grind leaves you with precious little time. But while your doctor may nod sympathetically upon hearing this excuse, your heart will be much less forgiving. If you don't have the time, make the time. Get up earlier, use the weekends more efficiently, make it your first priority after work, ideally before you get home. (Once we get home, most of us have a tough time finding our way to the gym.) Make it a ritual with your significant other.

The best cardio is the cardio you will actually do. As a goal, aim to achieve a heart rate of between 100 and 150 beats per minute for 30 to 45 minutes a day, 4 or 5 days week.

Give your doctor's office a quick call to let them know you're starting an exercise program. And let's not forget the simple things: just moving at all! It all adds up. You will feel better, look better, and sleep better, and your heart will thank you.

As we've said, if you take care of your heart, you may notice improvements in your overall health. And every change you make to benefit your heart will also benefit your brain. Let's dig a little deeper and find out exactly which 5-minute fixes will sharpen your thinking and keep you wise during those many extra years.

Chapter Three

Use Your Head

Our brains are marvels of evolution. Hidden within the folds of this little, 3-pound organ are vestiges of every one of our evolutionary predecessors. Like a farmhouse with new rooms added to accommodate an expanding family, our brains have sprouted new regions and lobes in response to the demands of our environment, allowing us to further grow and develop our abilities and skills over millennia. And while we might be highly intelligent beings with the ability to conceive of amazingly complex ideas like quantum physics, many of our day-to-day reactions and thoughts are still controlled by instincts for self-preservation that we've had since we crawled out of the swamp.

We've talked about that bittersweet irony of modern life, that many of the "advances" we created to make life easier are now threatening the very organ that dreamed them up! Luckily, we have the smarts we need to reverse that trend as well.

In the last chapter, we saw what a critical aspect of your well-being heart health is. But in order to have that heart pump—let alone to draw a breath, laugh, or make love—you have to have a strong and vital nervous system that is overseen by your own benevolent dictator, the brain.

Fix It in 5
Keep Your Brain Sharp

1. Do aerobic exercise, which increases brain-derived neurotrophic factor, a protein that protects and grows the brain.
2. Do resistance exercise, which helps to improve your body's insulin function, reducing damage to brain caused by high blood sugar.
3. Learn, read, take classes—challenge yourself!
4. Eat a diet rich in omega-3 fatty acids, fresh vegetables and fruits, and whole grains.
5. Watch less TV.

A 5-Minute Tour of Your Brain

We could write an entire library of books on the functioning of the nervous system, but its main function boils down to one thing: communication. The brain bellows commands from its perch inside our heads, using the spinal cord and nerves to transmit messages to every part of our bodies. Messages like "walk," "laugh," and "speak" are generated and controlled by the brain—not to mention the experiences of feeling sad while watching a movie, being inspired by a work of art, and deciding what to eat for dinner. The system that transmits that message up to the brain involves specialized, interconnected parts and substances—synapses, axons, dendrites, neurotransmitters, and the spinal cord itself—all working together like a relay team on a track to move chemical and electrical signals from even the most distant parts of the body up to the brain.

Divided into various regions, the parts of the brain are layered over one another, each one being responsible for performing specific tasks. Depending on the input, a message could go to many different parts of the brain for processing and reaction. Scientists believe the cerebrum, the largest, outermost part of the brain—the part that looks like a walnut—is the newest addition to the farmhouse of our brains, added most recently in the course of our evolution to control "higher level" thinking: intelligence, memory, personality, emotion, speech, and other complex tasks. The left side of the cerebrum tends to conduct analytical work—solving problems, applying logic, and making decisions— which is why we call people who love order, structure, and step-by-step processes "left brained." Meanwhile, the right side is responsible for creativity and our more typically "right-brained" activities—listening to music, creating art, and playing an instrument. Interestingly, the left part of the brain controls the right side of the body and vice versa— which may be why artists are more likely to be left-handed (and right-brained) than accountants are!

Think about the sheer complexity of the brain's tasks in a very simple encounter, like seeing a friend across the street. Your brain is sending tons of signals—"breathe," "blink," "turn head," "swallow," "shout," "wave hand," "watch and listen for cars," etc.—all simultaneously, all effortlessly. Amazing, isn't it? Every body function, every philosophical thought, is directed by the brain, while every input from the outside—smells, sights, other sensations—also builds new brain connections, helping in turn to mold the brain.

We're learning more each day about just how adaptable our brains are. But considering how critical the brain is for our survival, we're often quite cavalier about its daily care. So how can we lovingly care for it?

Feed It Well

This benevolent dictator is also somewhat of a resource hog. While the brain makes up less than 2 percent of the weight of your body, it consumes up to 20 percent of the calories you eat and 20 percent of the oxygen you breathe. Any health condition that prevents this vital nourishment from reaching the brain—such as high blood pressure or hardening of the arteries—can interfere with its ability to work. Over time, this chronic deprivation can starve the brain cells and even kill them, which experts believe is one of the contributing factors in cognitive decline. That's why anything that's good for the heart, anything that increases blood flow and enhances the body's ability to use oxygen and nutrients, is going to help your brain stay well fed and pleasantly plump.

Indeed, we love those fat brains. Healthy brains are actually two-thirds fat—but we're not talking deep-fried Oreo fat. No, our brains are quite discerning—they demand very special, "essential" fatty acids. The most critical of these are the omega-3s, which we discussed in Chapter 2. We can't make them within our bodies, so we have to get them from outside sources—and when you don't get enough, the very structure of your brain tissue can be compromised. Unfortunately, our modern diet has morphed to the point where we typically get only a small fraction of the amount of essential fatty acids we require—so getting plenty of omega-3s will be a major focus in our 5-minute fixes.

Give It a Rest

Like the heart, the brain never stops working—it's a 24/7 job to keep the body alive. But unlike the heart, the brain does grab a little downtime. After spending a full day frantically sending messages, our brains require roughly 8 hours to reboot. This doesn't mean that our brains shut down completely during sleep—in fact, sleep is a time of tremendous brain maintenance. Think of sleep as a time when the filing clerk in your brain organizes all the data you've collected during the day, storing memories and thoughts in the appropriate places, sweeping out the stresses of the day, and resetting the circulating levels of hormones and neurotransmitters so you'll be ready to tackle the next day's events. Like a cell phone charging overnight, sections of the brain, such as those responsible for decision making and emotions, take this chance to replenish their power supplies for the next day.

On the flip side, did you ever notice how sleep deprivation can turn us into hyperemotional basket cases? Without rest, the brain cannot continue working at full capacity. Reaction time and decision making are impaired as well (picture the nodding heads of drowsy drivers behind the wheel). Because of the importance of sleep, the brain creates a series of signals that force the body to prepare to close up shop for the night. When the sun goes down, your body temperature begins to drop and melatonin production kicks in, your eyes feel heavy, and your breathing slows down, and yep, this makes us feel like lying down.

Unfortunately, we may be addicted to using the original time-saver—artificial light— and caffeine to try to squeeze as much productivity and action into the day as we can. But these stimulants prevent the brain from switching into bedtime mode. And that lack of sleep can lead to elevated levels of stress hormones like cortisol. Heightened levels of cortisol have been shown to hamper memory and to literally decrease the size of the brain. So the next time you're tempted to stay up later to get more done, flip the switch instead. Dim the lights, stop working, and let your body do what it's designed to do. Sleep. Your brain will thank you for it.

Don't Be Afraid of Helmet Head

Considering the vital role that the brain plays in keeping the body alive, it's hard to believe it can be so fragile. Although it is encased in a protective layer of bone (the skull), the brain itself is a spongy, gelatinous organ with only fluid separating it from the skull. This setup may protect the brain from a bump on the head, but a more powerful whack or shake can seriously injure the brain and affect memory, speech, and balance and even cause bleeding in the brain. Protecting the developing brains of children and infants is important to prevent permanent, lifelong damage, but any jarring head strike or shake remains dangerous, no matter what your age.

WARNING SIGN! STROKE

Stroke is the third leading cause of death in America—so it's time for everyone to become an expert in detecting it, because every minute counts.

Be on the lookout for some of these warning signs of stroke—they can come on very quickly.

- Numbness in the face, arm, or leg
- Numbness primarily on one side of the body
- Difficulty seeing clearly, walking, and staying upright without support
- Dizziness
- Severe headache
- Confusion

If someone near you is experiencing anything like this, call 911 immediately—fast treatment with clot-busting drugs within the first 3 hours of a stroke is key to having the best outcome. You or your loved one might also be having a TIA—a transient ischemic attack, or "ministroke"—which is typically less damaging but indicates a higher risk of stroke in the future. Getting a prompt, proper diagnosis is essential to having a longer, happier life afterward.

Learn, Baby, Learn

When we are children, our brains are more elastic, making it easier for us to learn new things. Babies have 100 billion brain cells, but very few connections between those neurons. During the learning process, those neurons form trillions of connections.

WHAT YOUR BODY'S TRYING TO TELL YOU: HEAD INJURIES

We've heard some scary stories about head injuries in the news lately. Knowing the differences between everything from bumps and bruises to concussions and fractures can be very stressful, especially for parents of young kids. While we don't want you to panic, you should know that, in general, head injuries should be taken seriously—especially because they're hard to spot. This list can help you evaluate symptoms after a head injury so you know what to do next. (When in doubt, call your doctor or 911.)

Symptoms: Confusion, amnesia, headache, dizziness, ringing in the ears, nausea or vomiting, and slurred speech after the injury; in the hours or days after the injury, memory problems, sensitivity to light and noise, sleep problems, behavior changes (such as irritability, depression, or confusion), loss of smell or taste, balance problems
What it could mean: Concussion
What to do: Call your doctor right away. Children should see a doctor if they've gotten anything more than a light knock on the head.

Symptoms: Severe headache; dizziness; vomiting; unequal pupils; sudden weakness in an arm or leg; restlessness, agitation, or irritability; memory loss or forgetfulness
What it could mean: Contusion (bruised brain tissue)
What to do: Call your doctor right away. Get emergency help for anyone who loses consciousness or can't be awakened easily from sleep.

Symptoms: Bloody or clear fluid coming from the ears or nose, a headache that won't go away, persistent vomiting or nausea, convulsions, seizures, enlargement of one or both pupils, can't be awakened from sleep, trouble talking, weakness or numbness in the arms or legs, loss of coordination, behavioral changes such as confusion or agitation

Our brains make these connections, steadily adding to their number, and by age 3, a preschooler's brain has a quadrillion—that's 1,000 trillion—connections. By the time a child enters first grade, his or her brain will be 95 percent of its adult size, and it will continue to

What it could mean: Severe traumatic brain injury
What to do: Call 911 or go right to the emergency room.

Symptoms: Bleeding from a cut or gash on the head
What it could mean: Even minor cuts may bleed heavily
What to do: Apply pressure with a clean bandage or cloth for 20 minutes. (Don't apply pressure, however, if you think the skull may be fractured.) If the bleeding stops, apply an ice pack. Call 911 if bleeding is severe or won't stop after 20 minutes, or if any more serious symptoms appear.

Symptoms: Bleeding from a head wound or from the ears, the nose, or around the eyes; bruising behind the ears or under the eyes; unequal pupils; confusion, dizziness, headache, or loss of consciousness; stiff neck; swelling
What it could mean: Skull fracture (often invisible to an observer)
What to do: Call 911 immediately.

Symptoms: A bump or small bruise on the forehead
What it could mean: Harmless swelling or broken blood vessels from a minor bump on the head
What to do: Apply an ice pack wrapped in a towel (and keep watch for more serious symptoms listed in this chart). If condition worsens, contact a physician.

Symptoms: A small amount of blood coming from a cut or bump on the head
What it could mean: Just a minor cut (even small cuts can bleed a lot because there are lots of blood vessels in the head and face)
What to do: Wash, apply antibacterial ointment, and cover with a bandage if possible (and watch for more serious symptoms). If condition worsens, contact a physician.

steadily add gray matter until the age of 11 or 12. That's when the brain begins to "prune" less-used connections, allowing increasing specialization and focus (very often with a heavy emphasis on video game playing and skateboarding!).

Eventually, those connections will be pared down to those that are used most often and form everything from habits to taste preferences, from favorite sports to common patterns of thought in language and math. At first, this might be seen as a disaster—"Is my brain shrinking?"—until you realize that it is the pruning that allows more complex thought to develop.

Without your even telling your brain to do so, it clears out the unused connections like you would an overstuffed closet. Then, instead of risking tripping over last year's clothing, you're left with an easily accessible wardrobe that contains extremely versatile, ready-for-anything neural connections. That closet will serve you well for many years, especially if you make a concerted effort to keep challenging yourself mentally. Indeed, even though the number of neural connections decreases with age, you can actually be a much more nimble thinker because you bring tremendous perspective and a sense of history—what's worked and what hasn't—to each decision. Sure sounds like wisdom to us!

Researchers used to believe that, as we age, our nerve cells age as well and the signals they produce or transmit are slowed down, muddied, or stopped altogether—and, unfortunately, this can happen sometimes. Diseases like Alzheimer's can cause nerve cells or nerve messaging pathways to stop working, which can disrupt the delivery of important messages and result in memory loss, disorientation, and confusion. But luckily, in the past few years we've learned a tremendous amount about how the brain, when confronted with novel experiences, is actually incredibly malleable and has the ability to grow and change throughout the lifetime. And the process of tapping into that "neuroplasticity" is not only fun—and addictive!—it's as easy as taking 5.

5-Minute Fixes
for a Lifetime of Brain Health

When we looked at the studies of exceptional aging, we found near universal agreement: A long life is really only enjoyable when you can enjoy it! The presence of cognitive decline or Alzheimer's not only accelerates aging, but also decreases the quality of those remaining years. So the primary objective for our fixes here is to do everything we can to prevent that cognitive decline and turn back the hands on that aging clock, 5 minutes (or less!) at a time.

Unwrap a stick of gum before you do your taxes. A study published in the journal *Nutritional Neuroscience* found that chewing gum can actually sharpen your thinking. Researchers tested 133 people—half of whom were given mint-flavored gum and the other half, fruit-flavored gum—and subjected them to mental tests in both stressful and calm settings. When they chewed gum, they were more alert and happier and their reaction times were quicker. In fact, when they chewed gum, their reaction times got faster as the tasks became more difficult. Chewing gum also improved their ability to focus on one activity for longer periods of time—all of which can help you power through unpleasant but mentally challenging tasks more quickly, like doing your taxes. (No word came back on whether the fruit-flavored gum gets rid of the bad taste in your mouth afterward, though.)

Look for gum with the American Dental Association Seal of Acceptance. Rigorous standards set by this designation suggest that these brands may also help you prevent cavities, strengthen your teeth, and reduce harmful plaque. **Time spent:** 1 minute to find gum with the ADA Seal at the store and 10 seconds to unwrap a stick

Snack on a can of kippered fish (aka smoked herring). A serving of this deep-sea fish can pack more than 1.5 grams of the omega-3 fatty acids known to slow down plaque growth in arteries, reduce triglycerides, and lower the risk of abnormal heart rhythms. All of this without

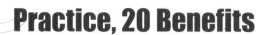

Practice, 20 Benefits
Mindfulness Meditation

On the whole, we humans are often in autopilot mode, moving quickly through our lives and our to-do lists without paying real attention to much of anything. Mindfulness meditation is a way of training your brain to notice and appreciate the details of your present experience, so you can really get the most out of the pleasurable moments of your life—and garner some significant health benefits while you're at it.

People can be very intimidated by the practice, but mindfulness meditation is actually very simple—you just sit quietly with your eyes closed and pay attention to an aspect of your current experience, focusing on one item at a time. You might start by noticing the flow of air in and out of your nostrils or your belly rising and falling with each breath. When you get distracted—and you will!—simply acknowledge the thought and turn your attention back to your breath

(or whatever it is that you're attending to).

This is the entire practice—you don't need any additional mental exercises. Simply reminding yourself to return your attention to your breath is what mindfulness is all about. That's the beauty of it! So simple. You might need to redirect yourself hundreds of times within a 5-minute period. Every time you do, it's like doing a mental pushup—you're making your brain stronger.

We'll admit, this is trickier than it sounds—we tend to get distracted by every little thought that comes into our heads: "It's too hot." "Did I pay that bill?" "What are we having for dinner?" The practice of mindfulness meditation will gradually help quiet that internal chatter, so your brain can tune in and be present in your life.

If that all sounds a bit woo-woo, we want you to know that you don't need to be a monk or hide out in a monastery—indeed, mindful-

the troubling worries over mercury and other heavy metals that accumulate in fish. (Herring are so low on the food chain that troublesome levels of these metals don't have a chance to accumulate in their bodies.)

Grab can, pull tab. Pair it with a slice of whole wheat toast and an apple or a tangerine for a fast lunch full of brainfood. **Time spent:** 20 seconds to open the can, 5 minutes to savor and enjoy

Put your head down at 2:00 p.m. A new study from the University of California at Berkeley

ness meditation is not affiliated with any religion. The practice has been extensively researched in clinical settings for many years—more than 20,000 studies, reviews, and papers examining some aspect of mindfulness are listed in the National Institutes of Health's National Library of Medicine. Many of them have found that, with long-term use, this simple process can yield tremendous physical, mental, and emotional health benefits with no discernible negative side effects. Even with just 5 minutes a day, you will start to see some improvements. This research suggests that mindfulness meditation may:

1. Reduce levels of chronic stress
2. Reduce pain
3. Lower cortisol, a stress hormone linked to early cognitive decline
4. Improve functioning of the adrenal glands
5. Lower heart and respiratory rates
6. Lower blood pressure
7. Lessen insomnia due to excessive worry
8. Enhance immune system function
9. Improve antibody response to flu vaccine
10. Increase energy
11. Reduce gastrointestinal upset
12. Relieve anger, depression, and anxiety
13. Reduce repetitive, ruminating thoughts
14. Increase empathy for oneself and others
15. Improve attention and ability to stay on task
16. Reduce judgmental thinking
17. Enhance the ability to quickly refocus after being distracted
18. Thicken the cerebral cortex, the brain region linked to planning and regulating emotions
19. Reduce automatic emotional reactivity (such as angry outbursts or anxiety attacks)
20. Increase your gray matter and grow the size of the brain (literally!)

People from all walks of life do mindfulness meditation. Even with just 5 minutes of practice a day, you will start to see some improvements. Now that's an excellent health fix if we've ever heard one.

determined that taking a 90-minute nap from 2:00 to 3:30 p.m. can increase your brain's ability to learn new information at 6:00 p.m. Turns out that during the stage 2 non-REM portion of your nap—the deep sleep that starts about 30 minutes after you first drift off—your brain takes facts and other information sitting in temporary storage in your hippocampus and refiles them in the prefrontal cortex for longer-term storage.

If you can push nap time a little bit longer, to 2 hours, you may reinforce the learning you did before you fell asleep. A Harvard study found that people who were taught a new skill before falling asleep could perform it better upon awakening than those who did not nap at all. The catch: You have to dream to get this benefit, and REM sleep doesn't start until about 90 minutes into your nap.

Either way, researchers believe that these results hint that a biphasic sleep schedule—sleeping twice during each 24-hour period—might actually make you smarter! And, by extension, sleep deprivation might make you stupider: If you stay awake overnight to cram for a presentation or an exam, your ability to absorb new information plummets by 40 percent because your brain so desperately wants to sleep. So don't do it. Take a siesta instead! **Time spent:** 90 to 120 glorious, relaxing minutes a day

Drive your car exactly 1 mile from your house. If you don't have somewhere to go such as the gym or a track, here is a simple, free tip: Choose a route that takes you along a pretty side road with sidewalks. Once the odometer reads exactly 1 mile, look out the window for a landmark—that's your goal.

Now, drive home, set the timer on your watch, and walk out the door. Try to get to that landmark in less than 20 minutes. Once you're there, set your timer again and head home.

Do this just three times a week, and you can lower your risk of stroke substantially. Researchers at the Harvard School of Public Health studied the exercise habits of almost 40,000 women and found that those whose walks netted them 2 miles in 40 minutes—a pace of 3 miles per hour—lowered their risk of stroke by 37 percent. And if a woman got in 120 minutes of walking each week—at any speed—she cut her risk by 30 percent. By walking that much that quickly, you'll cover all of your stroke-prevention bases in the minimum amount of time. **Time spent:** 5 minutes to map the route and call a friend to join you, plus 40 minutes three times a week

Or cut the route in half. Is 2 miles too far? Just cut it in half: Measure half a mile, get there in 10 minutes, get back in 10 minutes, and do it six times a week. Same result with more convenience. In a *JAMA* study, those who exercised for 142 minutes a week for 6 months enjoyed enhanced memory at the end of the study, an effect that stuck with them for an additional 12 months after they stopped exercising. (Talk about a good time investment!)

The researchers believe the effect was due to enhanced blood flow and brand-new brain connections created during exercise. **Time spent:** 3 minutes to map the route, then 20 minutes six times a week

Pop an aspirin (after you ask your doctor). Aspirin is not only an incredibly inexpensive anti-inflammatory that thins your blood by reducing the clumping of platelets in your arteries to lessen the risk of stroke, it may also help you think, speak, and react faster. A recent German study in the journal *Neurology* found that C-reactive protein, or CRP, a measure of inflammation in the blood, is also linked with problems with executive thinking skills. The frontal lobes of people with high levels of CRP appeared, on a structural level, to be 12 years older than those of people with the lowest levels. People with the highest measures of inflammation took almost 10 percent longer to complete tests of verbal memory, word fluency, and reaction time. The researchers stated that aspirin therapy might be helpful in lowering levels of CRP.

Check with your doctor to see if aspirin therapy might be right for you. If you're a woman approaching 65 or beyond, it can be especially useful in preventing stroke and reducing other cardiovascular disease risks. **Time spent:** 10 seconds (once you get the bottle open)

Eat four walnuts a day, especially if you're a vegetarian. An Italian study found that eating just a few walnuts a day may significantly increase your blood levels of essential fatty acids and can reduce your risk of stroke. This daily portion of walnuts doubled the participants' blood levels of alpha-linolenic acid (ALA), an omega-3 fatty acid found primarily in walnuts and other vegetarian sources such as flaxseed. Unlike omega-3s from animal sources, ALA has to be converted into eicosapentaenoic acid (EPA) and docosahexaenoic acid (DHA) in order to be used—which has always been a bit of a hassle for vegetarians, who can't benefit from the abundant, immediately available EPA and DHA in fish and fish oil and have to seek out extra sources of ALA as a result. But here's the amazing part: Eating four walnuts a day also tripled the amount of EPA in the body—making it an incredibly potent means of getting the fats most essential for brain health and stroke prevention.

Increasing your intake of walnuts can improve the function of your blood vessels, reduce your LDL levels, and relieve systemic inflammation, all of which decrease your risk of cognitive decline. In fact, this effect is practically instantaneous. If you have high cholesterol and you eat a really fatty meal—we're talking 80 grams of fat—a Spanish study found that eating just ⅓ cup of walnuts can immediately lower your blood pressure and increase blood flow by 24 percent. The fat and protein in walnuts make them especially satisfying, too. Be sure to choose raw and unsalted, and try to find organic. **Time spent:** 1 to 5 minutes to savor your delicious snack

Boot up your computer. In a small study of 24 people ages 55 to 76, UCLA researchers found that just doing Google searches and browsing the Web for an hour a day stimulates regions of the brain that control decision making, complex reasoning, and vision, such as the frontal lobe, anterior temporal region, anterior and posterior cingulate cortexes, and hippocampus. Those who had more experience with Internet searching showed more than twice as much brain activity as those who were 'Net novices. If you've never spent time on the Web, now's the time to start: Take a class at your local library, community college, or senior center, or have a computer-savvy loved one show you how to search for long-lost friends on Facebook. Connecting with people, whether in person or online, is another way to challenge your brain and keep it nimble. **Time spent:** 2 minutes to get online—where you take it from there is up to you!

Stand up while you surf (or watch TV). Of course, many people are the opposite of the online novices mentioned above—they might spend hours sitting in front of a computer or television screen. If you're an Internet addict, don't use the prior tip as an excuse to up your screen time. A recent study published in the journal *Circulation* followed 8,000 people in Australia and found that every hour of television watching per day increased their risk of dying from all causes by 11 percent and from cardiovascular diseases by a whopping 18 percent. Even those who had no previous cardiovascular disease and ate right and exercised experienced the same effect.

Head off some of these dangerous risks by creating a standing desk: Put your laptop on a pile of books on the counter or move the couch away from the TV and put a treadmill or stationary bike in its place. Or have a standing desk set up in your office, like Donald Rumsfeld. A computer can help your brain—but only if your body doesn't pay the price instead. **Time spent:** a few seconds to stand up—you're there anyway!

Take six deep breaths. Many of us have lives that feel like roller coasters—our stress level can be really high for a few weeks, but then it calms down for a while before it shoots up again. But even if your "normal" blood pressure is in the average range, that occasional blood pressure spike might be putting you at an increased risk for stroke. A study published in *The Lancet* found that people's peak blood pressures were better predictors of stroke than their average levels. Researchers reviewed the records of former TIA patients and found that those with the most-variable systolic pressure over the last seven visits to the doctor were six times more likely to have a stroke than those who had more stable blood pressure.

Don't fret, it's fixable. Making a conscious effort to calm yourself down during high-stress moments can help you manage these blood pressure surges. One Japanese study of more than 20,000 people found that taking six deep breaths in 30 seconds can drop your systolic blood pressure by up to 9.6 mmHg in people with hypertension and 6.4 mmHg for people with normal blood pressure. You might think about continuing this practice several times during the day, every day, for a speedy head-clearer with immediate benefits. **Time spent:** 30 seconds

Pump up the tires on your bike. A German study found that people who rode their bikes three times a week for 30 minutes each over a span of 3 months increased the volume of the hippocampus, a brain region associated with spatial navigation and long-term memory, by 16 percent. Researchers also found improvements in short-term memory. If you haven't broken out your wheels in a while, now's the time. Riding your bike around town is also a great way to mentally challenge your brain—you have to recall the best route to your destination, navigate narrow alleyways, and react to potholes—all of which push your brain to work in ways it normally might not during your everyday life. You'll burn calories, decrease your carbon footprint guilt, and likely run into a neighbor or two along the way—all good things for your

WHAT YOUR BODY'S TRYING TO TELL YOU: FORGETFULNESS OR ALZHEIMER'S?

Being afraid that we're losing our marbles is one of the most common concerns we feel as we're getting older. If this sounds like you, you might be reassured to learn that the people who forget things and worry about it typically are in better shape than those who don't worry about it at all—sadly, as cognitive decline advances, you're more likely to lose insight into your own abilities (or lack thereof).

Neurologists sometimes put it this way: It's not a problem when you forget where you put your keys; the problem comes when you forget what keys are for.

General signs deserving concern:

- Completely forgetting that you made an appointment, even when you've been reminded (not simply forgetting to go)
- Completely forgetting how (and why) to take your medication (not simply forgetting to take it)
- Completely forgetting how to get home from familiar places (not simply getting lost in unfamiliar territory)
- Completely forgetting that you just told someone a particular story and repeating the entire thing again (not simply losing track of what you've said when you're telling the story for the first time)

Here's the difference: Normal forgetfulness is the product of divided attention—if you were truly focused on what you were doing, you would not have made the error. But it's a sign of trouble when you are not even conscious that you made an error at all.

brain. Give your tires a pumping up and hit the streets. **Time spent:** 5 minutes to pump up the tires, then 30 minutes three times a week

Peel a banana. As you get older, if your blood pressure heads north of 140/90, your risk of developing brain lesions gets higher. These lesions have been linked with an increased risk of dementia. Tiny blood vessels that feed the white matter in your brain—60 percent of its total volume—are especially sensitive to any increase in blood pressure. The resulting lesions can disrupt communication between different regions of the brain. But research shows that you can start to reduce your blood pressure within 2 weeks of starting the DASH diet—short for Dietary Approaches to Stop Hypertension—recommended by the National Heart, Lung, and Blood Institute and the American Heart Association. On it, you'll avoid fat, salt, sugar, and cholesterol-rich foods and eat more low-fat dairy products, whole grains, fruits, and veggies. You'll also strive for 3,500 mg of dietary potassium a day, which you can get from broccoli (505 mg per cup), spinach (838 mg per cup), cantaloupe (494 mg per cup), and bananas (467 mg each). For more information about the DASH diet, check out www.dashdiet.org. **Time spent:** 30 seconds to peel and eat

Drop and give yourself 20. While we recommend doing plenty of aerobic exercise, which is critical to reducing blood pressure and increasing blood flow, we also hope you fit in some resistance exercise. A Canadian study of women ages 65 to 75 found that those who did resistance exercise just once a week enjoyed an enhanced ability to focus attention on a task, as well as a better aptitude for conflict resolution—which probably made them more fun to be around!

You don't have to belong to a gym to get a brain-boosting dose of resistance training. Instead, use your own body weight. Do as many pushups as you can during commercials, adding an extra two to five to each session as you gain strength. Lunge across the living room as you water plants or vacuum the carpet. If you have one, lift your baby above your head like a baby bench press. The trick is to challenge your muscles as much as you can as often as you can while you go about your daily life. **Time spent:** zero extra minutes, if you fit each into another daily activity

Sign up for yoga—for you and your kid. You don't have to be a die-hard yogi to get the brain-boosting benefits of one of the world's oldest stress-reduction techniques. You don't even have to be an adult! One study compared kids between 11 and 16 years old who attended a yoga camp, a fine arts camp, or neither. All were assessed at the start of camp and retested 10 days later. At the final assessment, the yoga group got significantly higher—by 43 percent—scores on spatial memory tests than the children who attended fine arts camp or just stayed home. Researchers credited the yogic breathing, meditation, and guided relaxation for the changes. Another study suggested that regular yoga practice can reduce the body's levels of the cytokine interleukin-6 (IL-6). "Huh?" you say. "What's that?" It's a marker for inflammation that's been linked to stroke, heart disease, diabetes, and other age-related diseases. Not only did regular yoga practitioners have lower amounts of IL-6 at the start of the study, but their levels of it also rose only slightly compared with the jumps in the yoga novices.

Time spent: either 5 to 10 minutes a day or a 30- to 40-minute session twice a week

Toss your bottled dressing and whip up this simple vinaigrette. A recent study published in the journal *Archives of Neurology* found that eating a diet rich in a combination of certain foods can decrease the risk of developing Alzheimer's by almost 40 percent. The researchers watched the diets of more than 2,000 New Yorkers ages 65 and up for about 4 years. They found that those who ate more olive-oil-based salad dressings, nuts, fish, tomatoes, poultry, fruits, and cruciferous and dark green leafy vegetables and mostly stayed away from red and organ meats and high-fat dairy products had the healthiest brains. Researchers believe this combination of nutrients may work together synergistically to protect both the heart and the brain, making it extra-effective in fending off cognitive decline.

With this all-star nutritional lineup of simple, whole foods, the only way you could go wrong in following this diet would be to use store-bought salad dressings, which can have a lot of fillers and thickeners—i.e., crap. To make it easy, buy a salad dressing mixing bottle from your grocer's kitchenware aisle and whip together the ingredients to make this very simple vinaigrette.

3   tablespoons balsamic vinegar
2   tablespoons extra virgin olive oil
½   clove garlic, minced
⅛   teaspoon dried basil
1   teaspoon salt
1   teaspoon ground black pepper

Splurge on high-end oil and vinegar—there's a huge taste difference. You'll want to have enough on hand so you never again give in to the premade-dressing time-saving temptation.

Time spent: 5 minutes preparing a batch to use for several days

Play an hour of Wii. A recent Canadian study found that playing games on Nintendo's Wii may actually help people recover their motor skills after a stroke—which hints that it may have positive benefits for everyone. Researchers compared two groups of stroke survivors between 41 and 83 years old who were in rehab. One group's members played recreational games like cards and Jenga, while the other's members played Wii Tennis or Wii Cooking Mama (a game that simulates doing kitchen work like shredding cheese and peeling an onion). After 2 weeks, the Wii group had significant improvement in their motor skills—they were 30 percent faster on a motor function test and had regained more of the abilities they'd lost, both in large body movement and fine motor skills—compared with the other group. Researchers believe the highly repetitive nature of the very specific tasks activated special brain cells called mirror neurons, which help us mimic others when learning and help our bodies remember how to perform certain actions. All of these results point to Wii's potential for helping our brains change and grow. Who would've thought it, huh? After all the time we've spent telling our kids, "Those video games will rot your brain!" **Time spent:** 60 fun minutes a day a few times a week

Ask yourself a hard question. To zero in on your life purpose, ask yourself, "If I could change one thing about the world, what would it be?" In a recent study published in the *Archives of General Psychiatry,* researchers spoke with 900 older folks living in senior housing and found that the ones who claimed to have a strong "purpose in life" were two and a half times more likely to ward off Alzheimer's or its precursor, mild cognitive impairment.

Not only may having a clear life purpose protect your brain's health when you get older, it can also improve your life today—people who commit themselves to goal-directed activities

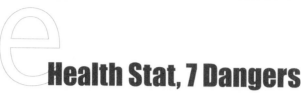

Health Stat, 7 Dangers
Waistline Measurement

Recent research from the University of Southern California in Los Angeles found that women between the ages of 35 and 64 have three times the risk of stroke as men of the same age. Perhaps the biggest risk factor? That roll around the middle.

Guys tend to know their approximate waist measurement because that's how they buy their pants. But the average woman can float along for years in a fog, happily imprecise about her waist stat. Sadly, that ignorance is not bliss for the brain. In comparison to almost any other health indicator, our waist measurement tells us a whole constellation of bad stuff might be going on inside. While middle-aged women generally enjoy healthier cholesterol levels and lower blood pressure than men do, their belly fat can set them up for other potentially dangerous conditions that all but negate those positive health factors.

Once a woman's waist measures more than 35 inches (or a guy's waist is bigger than 40 inches), risks dramatically rise for:

1. stroke (a 400 percent increase!)

tend to be more social and outgoing, less depressed and anxious—all good things for brain health. And being a part of something larger than yourself is one of the most powerful happiness habits there is.

Answer the "If I could change one thing about the world, what would it be?" question quickly, with your first instinctive reaction. Then take some more thoughtful time to brainstorm five different ways to contribute to making that change on a local level, whether by volunteering at your local school or hospital, writing letters to your government representatives, or canvassing door-to-door for a local campaign you believe in. When you're done making your list, circle the action you're most interested in and make one call—to campaign headquarters, the animal shelter, the United Way office—that will get you one step closer to getting

2. cardiovascular disease

3. type 2 diabetes

4. high blood pressure

5. heart failure

6. systemic inflammation

7. asthma

So if you've put on a few, rather than focusing on pounds, make whittling those waistline inches your top priority. Even in a woman of normal weight, an increase of 4 inches in the waist over the years raises her risk of heart failure by 15 percent compared with women whose waist sizes stay the same. And if you tend to manage your weight by dieting instead of exercising, you may be "skinny fat"—your frame may be slender but metabolically active fat may be lurking inside, surrounding your internal organs. If you are of normal weight but basically sedentary, body composition may be more appropriate for you to determine your level of risk—and stepping up your activity level will greatly reduce your risks of disease.

For most of us, though, a simple waist measurement will speak volumes. Wrap a tape measure around your belly, directly across your navel, and note your measurement. Repeat once a week, tracking your changes. (One note: Don't get alarmed if you jump up a few inches during your period—it happens to everyone!) Keep reminding yourself of the bonuses that come with less belly: More energy, easier breathing, less bathing suit anxiety, cuter clothes—and even belts!

involved. **Time spent:** 20 seconds to ask the question, 5 minutes to brainstorm activities linked to your purpose, 5 more minutes to make the first call

Wash your hands. Okay, we all know that having a cold sore is pretty gross. But you might be surprised to learn that what's a tiny nuisance now could be a sign you're at risk for Alzheimer's. A recent Canadian review of studies involving certain pathogens, including herpes simplex virus type 1, picornavirus (the family of viruses that cause everything from the common cold to polio), and *Helicobacter pylori* (the bacterium that causes stomach ulcers) along with several others, found that systemwide infections may impact the central nervous system and possibly contribute to the development of cognitive decline or even Alzheimer's. If you've had chronic problems with infections from any pathogen, take extra care to safeguard your immune system with simple, commonsense hygiene. Be sure to wash your hands thoroughly after using the toilet, sneezing, or touching surfaces that have been touched by many others—handrails on escalators, a hang strap on the subway, a public phone. Avoid antibacterial soaps that include triclosan, a chemical that may interfere with your body's normal hormonal balance as well as lead to antibiotic resistance. Because superbugs are on the rise, you might also consider bolstering your body's defenses with the "good" bacteria in probiotic capsules that aid digestion to help crowd out errant invaders before they can get a foothold in your body. **Time spent:** 2 minutes every time you wash

Clear off the table. And pull the sticky notes off your computer. And file that pile of papers. It turns out that the same clutter that is a distracting nuisance to most of us could be downright painful to people who get migraines. Scottish researchers studied the effect of "visual noise" on people who suffered from regular migraines. When compared with folks who didn't get migraines, those who did were more likely to have trouble searching for and pinpointing a specific object when it was surrounded by other visual distractions. The clutter might even provoke migraines by triggering whole clusters of nerve cells to become overactive, just like a muscle spasm.

Cutting the clutter not only helps migraine sufferers, it relieves stress for everyone, helping you focus your attention by allowing you to consider one thing at a time and increasing your sense of calm. Don't beat yourself up if your house doesn't look like Martha Stewart's or the ones in *Real Simple*—whose does?—but build in those microbursts of straightening up a little bit every day. Pick two times of the day that mess usually accumulates. And go for it. It will save you a big headache later! **Time spent:** 2 to 3 minutes once or twice a day

Drs' Orders

for Nervous System Health: Sleep 7 Hours a Night

Everything falls apart when we don't sleep: We get cranky and short-tempered, we make goofy mistakes in our work, we eat more poor-quality foods, we don't exercise enough. People who sleep less than 5 hours a night can even gain up to 32 percent more fat, all of it packed into the belly, forming that toxic belly fat that can all but suffocate those vital organs. When study participants who were allowed to sleep less than 6.5 hours were compared with those whom the researchers let sleep for more than 7.5 hours, the short sleepers were found to have developed insulin resistance—the reduced ability of the body to lower a blood sugar increase caused by eating and frequently a predecessor of diabetes—in just 8 days!

But just think about how great you feel when you do get enough sleep. You feel more patient and compassionate, less reactive to bad behavior. Your skin glows from the restorative rest. You have more energy for your life, whether you need it for chasing your rug rats or chasing your ideal bottom line. Sleep is your brain's best friend.

Starting now, you're going to make sleep a priority. Remove the television, laptop, snoring dogs, extra work, clutter—everything that makes your bedroom a less than tranquil sanctuary. Avoid having more than one alcoholic drink before bed; contrary to popular belief, alcohol actually stimulates your body rather than relaxes it. Set a bedtime and a wake-up time, take a shower or bath before bed, and put a worry book on your nightstand for capturing those 2:00 a.m. frets. But more than anything, just go to bed! Your life will still be there in the morning. And since you'll be properly refreshed and rejuvenated, you'll greet it with a wide smile and a deep, cleansing breath—which is the topic of our very next chapter.

Chapter Four
Breathe Easy

Taking a deep breath is one of life's most pleasurable small acts. We can go through our entire day without ever really zeroing in on this automatic process, while every breath brings in one of the 10,000 smells the average human being is capable of recognizing—a fresh cup of coffee, a baby's sweet skin, the scent of spring flowers. Small patches of nerve cells, called olfactory sensory neurons, connect directly to the brain, and each of these neurons has one odor receptor stimulated by certain scents. When tiny molecules are released into the air as flowers bloom, the precise combination of those triggered receptors register as "the smell of daffodils."

For some, those spring flowers are an olfactory delight; for others who have environmental allergies, they wreak havoc. From smoke to exhaust fumes to gases emitted by new carpets, our bodies instinctively recoil from scents that are toxic. That instinct to hold our noses acts as our own canary in the coal mine—and we should pay close attention to it. But if we take a moment each day to appreciate our breath and all it brings to us, we'll not only be more aware of how to protect our airways from potential dangers, we'll also smell more of those delightful scents that make life so much richer.

Fix It in 5
Keep Your Lungs Clear

1. Don't smoke!
2. Reduce your exposure to environmental toxins (from car exhaust, industrial cleaners, pesticides, paints, air freshners, and so on).
3. Keep your stress level low.
4. Use air-conditioning, filtration systems, and houseplants to clean indoor air.
5. Avoid known allergens, such as dust mites and excess pollen, as much as possible.

A 5-Minute Tour of Your Lungs

In the next minute, you will take between 15 and 20 breaths. In the next 24 hours, 25,000. You don't have to think about your respiratory system in order to use it, but this delicate system is responsible for bringing life-giving oxygen to your entire body.

When you inhale air, your diaphragm—a large, flat muscle stretched out at the bottom of your lungs—contracts and your rib muscles lift the rib cage up to allow room for the lungs to fill. As the air travels from your nose and mouth and down your trachea, it passes tiny hairs called cilia, which hopefully filter out junk like dust or pollen that has traveled in with the air. After passing through this filtering system, the air enters the lungs—and once it gets there, that air has some room to play in. The surface area of the lungs is about the size of a tennis court!

An unbelievable 600 million alveoli (no, guys, not areolae, the area around the nipples—they're the tiny air sacs in your lungs) absorb the air, grab the oxygen, and hand it over to blood cells that are passing through on their way back to the heart. The heart then pumps those oxygen-filled blood cells throughout the body. As the next shipment of blood leaves the lungs bound for the heart, the "used" blood enters the lungs and deposits carbon dioxide waste in the alveoli to be exhaled through the mouth and nose. Amazing, right? Our bodies are the original recycling plants, efficiently taking used blood and turning it right around for our bodies to use to move about during our day without even thinking about it.

Cough It Up

While the body has filters in place to remove junk from the air you breathe, certain things like pollution and cigarette smoke are no match for them. Your body has a very exotic backup defense system to get rid of particles that we inhale—it's called coughing. When viruses, bacteria, smoke, or other particulates get into the airways, they cause an irritating tickle that makes the muscles contract to generate a cough. The goal of coughing is to expel the particles up the airway and out through the mouth—which is why it's not always a good idea to suppress a cough with drugs (despite the dirty looks your co-workers are giving you).

Considering how much our lungs don't like extra stuff getting in them, it is baffling that so many people continue to smoke. Smoke compounds all of these issues with countless other problems. ("I'll see your chronic coughing and raise you addictive toxins!") Chemicals in cigarette smoke can cause the lungs to swell or destroy the lung tissue, making it difficult to breathe and all too often resulting in lung cancer. Or, smokers can develop chronic obstructive pulmonary disease, or COPD—a condition found most often in current or past smokers, whose airways and air sacs have lost their elasticity and become thick, inflamed, and full of mucus. People with COPD wheeze, feel short of breath, experience chest tightness, and cough up large amounts of slimy mucus. (Smoking is so glamorous, isn't it?)

Now, not everyone who suffers from these lung conditions is a smoker. Indeed, the poor kids and other bystanders who have to breathe in secondhand smoke are severely impacted by its thousands of toxic chemicals, including benzene, chromium, cyanide, formaldehyde, and lead. Oh, and polonium—you know, that radioactive poison sometimes used to kill spies.

And what about the toxic chemicals in air pollution? You may not be a smoker or even live with one, but industrial pollutants and unregulated chemicals in the environment or your broom closet are treating your body like an ashtray, risking your health in many of the same ways. You have to become conscious about how to avoid or minimize your contact with these pollutants—primarily by choosing natural home cleaners and personal care products, paints with low volatile organic compounds, and other safe products—and we'll show you how.

Many of these inhaled pollutants can greatly aggravate asthma—a condition in which the airways are swollen and sensitive that makes breathing laborious because air has to squeeze through narrowed passageways. Most people whose asthma is under control have many good days of relatively easy breathing and few problems. But even among those with very well-controlled asthma, "attacks" can strike. During these attacks, the extent of the swelling varies—some people can recover on their own by using a rescue inhaler, while others need medical attention to force open the airways. If you find yourself needing to use your inhaler more than twice a week, you're waking up at night because of breathing problems, or you experience symptoms at least once a day, it's time to visit the specialist and see what's up.

When you think about protecting your lungs, it's helpful to remember that lungs are sweet, vulnerable little organs with very few natural defenses. Their passageways are literally connected to the outside air, so if you're serious about protecting them, you have to go a little mama bear: Consider avoiding fragrance, and use natural cleaning products. Avoid strong fumes from paint and other household chemicals. Don't use bleach, scented laundry detergent, or dryer sheets. Keep your windows rolled up when you're stuck in stop-and-go traffic. Oh, yeah, we almost forgot—please don't smoke.

WHAT YOUR BODY'S TRYING TO TELL YOU: COUGHING AND WHEEZING

The next time you or someone you love coughs, pay attention. Every cough is trying to tell you something. Some are signs that you simply have a cold. Others are red flags signalling more serious health problems, like asthma. Here's how to tell them apart.

Symptom: Cough with a sore throat
What it could mean: Postnasal drip
What to do: Call the doctor if you have a fever, if the mucus you cough up has a foul smell, or if these symptoms last for longer than 10 days in a child who is younger than 3 years old or for longer than 3 weeks in older kids, teens, and adults.

Symptom: Cough that gets worse in cold weather, when you exercise, or at night
What it could mean: Asthma
What to do: See your doctor for an evaluation.

Symptom: Cough with heartburn
What it could mean: Gastrointestinal reflux disease (known as GERD)
What to do: Avoid GERD trigger foods (caffeine, chocolate, high-fat foods, acidic foods), eat more frequent but smaller meals, and don't lie down after eating. Over-the-counter antacids, proton pump inhibitors such as omeprazole (Prilosec) and esomeprazole (Nexium), and H2 receptor antagonists such as cimetidine (Tagamet) and ranitidine (Zantac) can help. See your doctor if symptoms don't improve in 2 to 3 weeks.

Symptom: Cough with runny nose, sore throat, and fatigue. May also have a fever; chest pain; hoarseness; crackling or whistling breath sounds; and phlegm that's clear, white, yellow, or green

Stand Clear

You may have spent most of your life believing the old wives' tale that cardio work "conditions" your lungs. Well, that's close to the truth, but not exactly correct. Unlike muscles, lungs don't get bigger or stronger from exercise, and, likewise, they don't shrink from lack of exercise. So, if you are out of shape and have trouble catching your breath during strenuous

What it could mean: Bronchitis
What to do: See your doctor right away if you have a high fever, feel very sick and weak, cough up blood, are short of breath, have a weakened immune system or COPD, or if symptoms don't go away within 2 weeks.

Symptom: Wheezing that comes on very suddenly in a child
What it could mean: A foreign object may be lodged in his or her windpipe
What to do: Call the doctor immediately if you suspect that something's stuck in your child's throat. Call 911 if your child is having difficulty breathing.

Symptom: Wheezing only at specific times of year (spring, summer, or fall, depending on where you live)
What it could mean: Pollen allergy
What to do: An over-the-counter or prescription allergy medicine could help. (Watch for wheezing with shortness of breath, a warning sign that it could be asthma instead of an allergy. Kids who wheeze should be evaluated by a doctor.)

Symptom: A "barking" cough and difficulty breathing that may be worse at night
What it could mean: Croup
What to do: Call your doctor right away for advice. Croup causes the airways in the lungs to swell and immediate care may be required. Often, however, using a cool-mist.vaporizer, taking a warmly dressed child out into the cool night air, or sitting in a steamy bathroom brings relief. Acetaminophen may make him or her more comfortable.

activity, don't blame your lungs. Here's what really happens: A body that is conditioned to exercise is able to more efficiently distribute oxygen from the lungs to the heart and to the muscles throughout the body. But healthy lungs are always capable of meeting the increased demand for oxygen, so if you condition the rest of your body with regular exercise, your lungs will be able to keep up. In other words, they will work as hard as you do, if you give them the chance.

Rest (Un)easy

We usually don't give breathing a second thought—it just keeps trucking along, minute after minute, year after year. But in some people, this automatic process gets disturbed in a scary way in the middle of the night—with sleep apnea. While the bed partners of those with sleep apnea might claim to be the greatest sufferers—"Can you please keep it down over there?"—sleep apnea can be physically devastating for those who have it. Sometimes even deadly.

More than 18 million American adults have sleep apnea. People who have sleep apnea stop breathing several times an hour throughout the night, which interrupts their sleep, deprives their bodies of oxygen, and leaves them tired and exhausted the next morning. The most common cause of sleep apnea is an obstructed airway due to either muscles along the airway collapsing and closing the trachea or fat pushing on the airways, narrowing them and making breathing laborious. As with so, so many other health concerns, if you are overweight and you have sleep apnea, your best first defense is—you guessed it—to lose weight. One Temple University study found that when people who were obese lost just 10 percent of their body weight, they experienced complete or almost complete relief from sleep apnea.

5-Minute Fixes
for a Lifetime of Lung Health

Lungs may be powerful enough to keep us alive, but they are also delicate and vulnerable. Tiny particles, clouds of toxins, and other dangerous substances can make their way directly from the environment into these critical organs—and interfere with your most basic body functions immediately. Our natural defenses usually can handle this, but we have to do what we can to protect our organs and our breathing, too.

The exceptional aging studies are clear: Without a doubt, the most important thing you can do to protect your lung health and your longevity is to quit smoking. But aside from this obvious one, you might be surprised by the other small steps you can take to safeguard these incredibly fragile and absolutely essential organs.

Pour a snack of high-fiber cereal. A study published in the *American Journal of Epidemiology* found that eating more fiber reduces the odds of developing COPD. The study followed 111,580 people over nearly 2 decades and found that the people who ate the most fiber (typically about 28 grams per day) had a 33 percent lower risk of COPD than the group that consumed the least fiber. When comparing the effects of the fiber in grains, fruits, and vegetables, they found that only fiber from grains was linked to COPD risk reduction. Researchers believe that grain fiber has antioxidant and anti-inflammatory properties that might help fend off lung disease.

Having a bowl of high-fiber cereal every morning is not only a great way to get those grains, but research also shows that this breakfast is one of the most reliable tools in any successful weight-loss program (and losing excess pounds will help ease breathing issues as well). Pack a zipper-lock bagful in your backpack, glove compartment, or purse; sneak it into the movie theater to snack on instead of popcorn. (We won't tell!) Train yourself to crunch on cereal instead of chips or other salty snacks and you'll easily blow past the minimum goal of eating 25 to 35 grams of fiber every day. **Time spent:** 10 seconds to pour a bowlful

Swap a beef burger for a veggie one. A Japanese study of roughly 75,000 men and women found that men who never smoked and ate the most soy had half the risk of lung cancer of nonsmokers who ate the least amount of soy. While soy's isoflavones might guard against lung cancer, the researchers noted that the risk reduction they observed could be attributable to other factors—in other words, men who eat soy might be more likely to eat more vegetables, exercise more, drink less, and so on. Given the controversies about soy's hormonal activities—it can simulate estrogen in the body—we caution you not to go overboard. Talk with your doctor about how much soy is right for you. Check the ingredient list on your veggie burger for soy— and if there are more than 10 ingredients, put them back in the freezer. (That level of processing pretty much voids any potential benefits of the veggie burger.)

One thing is certain—eating less meat will help us stay slim, avoid excess saturated fat, and reduce our carbon footprint. According to calculations from environmental policy writer Jamais Cascio, if we all commit to eating just one burger a week instead of the average three we do eat, the nation could spare the environment 130 million metric tons of carbon dioxide— and the further gunking up of our air! **Time spent:** 2 minutes to pick out a box at the store (the prep time's about the same for beef or veggie)

Take your medication at night. Often allergies are at their worst first thing in the morning, which can make a normal wake-up downright inhuman. If that's the case for you, it might be better for you to take your allergy medication at night. Many allergy medications cause drowsiness, so what better time to lay back, relax, and let the medication do its work? **Time spent:** 10 seconds

Fire up the Neti pot. Pouring warm salt water up your nose might sound like a tamer version of waterboarding, but using nasal irrigation as a benign solution to sinus woes has

My son's nose is always stuffed up. When he
talks, he sounds like he has nose plugs on.
Even when he blows his nose, it doesn't make
any difference. How can I help him?

Dr. Drew says . . .

It sounds like your son has rhinitis, an inflammation of the inside of the nose. The resulting congestion overstimulates the mucous glands and causes overproduction of normal
nasal secretions.

Ask your pediatrician for an allergy screen for your son. If that comes back clean, your
son may have nonallergic rhinitis, which can be triggered by changes in temperature and
weather, odors, certain foods, and other environmental factors. You could first try some
nondrug nasal irrigation, such as a saline nasal spray or Neti pot. You know how salt
absorbs water? Both of these saline methods draw the fluids out of the inner lining of your
nose toward the salt, so it can be flushed away. The Neti pot has the added benefit of
volume—imagine giving the inside of your nose a nice, refreshing shower that wipes away
all the excess snot and grime. (See more on Neti pots on page 74.)

Nonallergic rhinitis can also be treated with over-the-counter decongestants, but if
the problem continues after taking medication, he should see a doctor for more testing.
One thing you shouldn't do is ignore the issue: Inflammation can lead to nasal polyps,
which form inside the sinuses and nasal lining and require surgical removal.

been around for millennia in Ayurvedic medicine. This traditional treatment has been
enjoying a resurgence lately as anecdotal evidence accumulates that Neti pot use could help
you recover more quickly from a cold, flu, or acute sinus infection. If you find yourself
taking more antibiotics than you'd prefer and you'd prefer to take a more natural route, you
might want to try a Neti pot, available from your local pharmacy for less than $10, and

follow the package directions. To make your own Neti pot solution, Mayo Clinic experts recommend stirring salt into 8 ounces of distilled, filtered, or otherwise purified water. You can use boiled tap water, but the important thing is to reduce potentially harmful impurities like chlorine—which is, after all, bleach! Cool the water to room temperature, then add ⅛ teaspoon of noniodized salt, such as kosher or sea salt. Use a full Neti pot for each nostril. Lean over the sink, tilt your head to the side, and pour the saltwater into the nostril on the top to literally wash away allergens, mucus, and bacteria. Dr. Jim recommends talking as you pour to prevent yourself from breathing any liquid in. (See a video of Dr. Jim bravely trying this at www.thedoctorstv.com/main/procedure_list/130) **Time spent:** 2 minutes per nostril

Join an asthma support group. Smokers are not the only ones who struggle with emotional issues related to their respiratory health. Having asthma can also increase your risk of depression. A study published in the journal *Chest* found that people with asthma are twice as likely to experience depression or anxiety. But another study noted that people who belonged to a support group for asthma tended to stay more consistent with their treatment plans and draw great strength from others in the same boat. Ask your pulmonologist (lung specialist) for a recommendation—if you live in a big enough city, your local hospital may have an affiliated program. Or search online at www.lungusa.org for the nearest location of the American Lung Association's asthma support and education program, Breathe Well, Be Well. Once you're in the group, find a buddy to befriend whom you can speak with outside of group time. If you're a Facebook addict, start an online asthma support group for sharing information and for commiseration on rough days. Just reach out—with up to 34 million Americans diagnosed with asthma, you are not alone. **Time spent:** 5 minutes to search for and find a group in your area

Toss your plastic food containers. Research published in Environmental Health Perspectives and conducted on mice showed a link between bisphenol A (BPA) exposure and allergies. The mice exposed to the chemical, which is commonly used in making plastics, at a level similar to

I've just been to the doctor, and all my
test and blood work results looked fine.
If I'm still healthy now, why should I quit
smoking? Maybe I'm one of the lucky ones.

A study that tracked British doctors for more than 50 years found that those who smoked their entire lives died 10 years earlier than nonsmokers, those who stopped at 50 died 4 years earlier, and those who stopped at 30 avoided almost all risk of premature death. The longer you wait, the more likely you'll be to develop cancer or COPD, which will make your last years on earth pretty miserable. But if you stop now, according to the American Cancer Society, look where you could be:

- 20 minutes after quitting: Your heart rate and blood pressure drops.
- 12 hours after quitting: The carbon monoxide level in your blood returns to normal.
- 2 weeks to 3 months after quitting: Your circulation improves and your lung function increases.
- 1 to 9 months after quitting: Coughing and shortness of breath decrease; your cilia (tiny hairlike structures that move mucus) regain normal function in the lungs, increasing their ability to handle mucus, clean the lungs, and reduce the risk of infection.
- 1 year after quitting: Your excess risk of coronary heart disease is half that of a smoker.
- 5 to 15 years after quitting: Your stroke risk is reduced to that of a nonsmoker.
- 10 years after quitting: Your chance of dying from lung cancer will fall to about half that of a person who continues smoking. Your risk of cancers of the mouth, throat, esophagus, bladder, cervix, and pancreas decrease, too.
- 15 years after quitting: Your risk of coronary heart disease is the same as a nonsmoker's.

You don't have to stop smoking on your own. Get evaluated for how severe your addiction is and find out what's sucking you in and keeping you smoking. Get a screening for depression. Up to one-third of all smokers experience mood, anxiety, or depressive symptoms that trap them into feeling like they need nicotine.

—***Linda Hyder Ferry, MD,*** *associate professor,*
Preventive Medicine and Family Medicine, Loma Linda University School of Medicine

that of most American adults developed bronchial inflammation and a greater sensitivity to allergens than nonexposed mice. BPA is used in many plastics bottles and in the liners of most aluminum cans, and its use has been banned in Canada and Denmark due to its possible links to diabetes, breast cancer, obesity, miscarriage, and spontaneous birth defects. Researchers posit that BPA may be partly to blame for the increase in asthma and allergy rates in the United States.

If you've been hoarding old takeout containers, take 5 minutes to go through them. Recycle every one that bears a "7" or a "PC" (for "polycarbonate"). If you have a Nalgene brand water bottle, be sure it does not have the 7 or PC label—Nalgene stopped using BPA in 2008 in response to public outcry and the more than 100 studies that attributed some level of biological risk to it. Try to avoid canned foods, as practically every single can in America is lined with plastic that includes BPA, especially tomato products (because the tomato's acidity makes more BPA leach into the food). For a million reasons, repeat after us: Stay away from BPA! **Time spent:** 5 minutes to sort through the to-go containers

Do a quick vaccine locator search at www.flu.gov. Find the closest place to get a flu vaccine and call to put yourself on the list. The H1N1 vaccine will be included in the seasonal vaccine beginning in the fall of 2010 and for as long as necessary until the majority of the country gets immunity. Most doctors recommend getting it in October or November to ensure maximum coverage over the entire season.

In the H1N1 crisis in 2009, many patients survived the initial H1N1 infection only to be taken down by complications from a resulting secondary pneumonia—which also could have been prevented by a vaccine. Pneumonia is the leading cause of vaccine-preventable death in the United States, and luckily, pneumococcal shots are available anytime—so why not start building your immunity today? Talk to your health care provider to find out if the pneumonia vaccine is right for you. **Time spent:** 5 minutes to locate the closest vaccine provider and call for an appointment

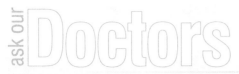

I've always heard that you should "starve a fever." Is that true?

Dr. Travis says . . .

Actually, the opposite is true—you should drown a fever. A fever is usually a sign of infection in the body, and you should be drinking plenty of fluids (not soda, folks!) to help prevent dehydration, especially if your fever is accompanied by vomiting and/or diarrhea.

Not only should you not starve a fever, you should instead fill your plate with disease-fighting foods like fruits and vegetables when you're sick—they're packed with antioxidants that strengthen your immune system and help you fight off your illness as fast as possible. The one thing I would recommend "starving" yourself of is sugar. White sugar and refined carbs inhibit your immune system—kind of the opposite of what you're going for, right?

Look for a company that does radon testing near you. We tend to run hot or cold with radon—we're very concerned about it when we're looking to buy a house, but then completely forget about it once we move in. But radon, the invisible gas that causes 3 to 14 percent of all cases of lung cancer, seeps through the cracks in the basements of many homes whose residents are completely oblivious. Don't wait until you put your house on the market to test for radon—protect your family now. You can buy self-testing kits (they run from $10 to $20) or call a professional (which will usually cost about $150 or more). If your home has a high radon level, it can be fixed. **Time spent:** 2 minutes to find and make the phone call, or 5 minutes to hang and then retrieve a radon self-test

Work it . . . in. While many of us think of winter as the prime gym season, for seasonal allergy sufferers, exercising outdoors in the pollen-heavy spring and summer seasons is way worse. You could be torturing your body unnecessarily if you work out outside—your increased respiratory rate as you huff and puff away draws in extra allergens. Having the air-conditioned comfort that a year-round gym membership provides can be a great investment in your health. Tear out all of the ads in your local newspaper that are for gyms within close driving distance. Then give each a call and start bargaining—many gyms give great deals during the "outdoor" months. (If you can't afford a gym membership, invest $10 in a new exercise DVD, or simply walk up and down the stairs of your house.) **Time spent:** 5 minutes to clip and save (your lungs)

Avoid scented candles. Scented candles tend to be one of those go-to solutions when something is smelling a little funky and last-minute guests stop by. Well, here's the thing—they don't actually "freshen" the air, they just mask odors. Plus, they can trigger asthma with their smoke, while also releasing volatile organic compounds into the air and adding extra perfumes and fragrances—which can also trigger attacks in many people. Minus the smoke factor, many of the same negatives apply to plug-in air fresheners, scented laundry and dish detergents, and dryer sheets. Some people are very sensitive to these scents and need to avoid them entirely; others can tolerate them. But perhaps the best, healthiest option is to figure out what is causing any stink you don't like in your house, then clean it up and ventilate to add fresh air.

Another option for stubborn odors or closed-up winter months: activated bamboo charcoal filters. Entirely nontoxic, these true air "fresheners"—they absorb odors from the air—can be used for many months, with just a quick shake needed every week to reactivate the charcoal. Do a search online; they're more expensive than candles and similar air fresheners, but they're totally green and last a long time. **Time spent:** 5 minutes to gather up the scented "fresheners" and toss them in the trash

Grab a local honey. Recent research has found that honey is a much more effective cough suppressant than most over-the-counter cough medicines, and without the extra unnecessary drugs. A bonus for allergy sufferers: Eating local honey (made by bees who live near the sources of your seasonal allergies) could stimulate your immune system and act as the equivalent of allergy shots. Natural health advocates all over the world have used this approach for centuries.

Seek out a honey producer within 10 miles of your home and ask for honey produced during the season when your allergies are the worst. The more natural (i.e., unrefined) the honey is, the better the immune response is thought to be. With the approval of your doctor, start taking a teaspoon three times a day or a tablespoon twice a day a month before your normal allergy season begins and track your symptoms—you might find relief quicker than you think. For added allergy-fighting potency, add pollen: Brew a tea with freeze-dried nettle leaves and add a teaspoon of local pollen and a teaspoon of local honey (all available at your local health food store).

If you or your child is struggling with a cough, take this opportunity to boost your immunity with local honey in this homemade cough medicine (otherwise known as an oxymel) specially prepared for us by natural health expert Chris Kleronomos, DAOM, FNP. (Note: Due to their immature immune systems, babies under 1 year old should not ingest honey.)

INGREDIENTS

- 32 ounces raw honey
- 3 ounces dried ginger root
- 8 ounces apple cider vinegar (look for unpasteurized and unfiltered brands with beneficial probiotic "live mother culture," such as Eden Organic)
- 1 tablespoon ground cinnamon
- 1 tablespoon propolis

DIRECTIONS

1. Place the honey in a medium bowl.
2. Shred and crush the ginger and add it to the honey.
3. Seal and let it stand for 24 hours.
4. Strain the mixture.

Continued

5. Pour the vinegar into a separate bowl, then add the cinnamon and stir until it has dissolved.
6. Add the vinegar mixture to the honey mixture and stir until well combined, and then stir in the propolis.

Store it in a tightly sealed glass jar, where it will keep indefinitely. (Just watch for green or black moldy growth, foul odor, or slimy material on top; but otherwise, rest assured—honey does not go bad.) Children and adults can take 1 tablespoon up to four times daily. Or just grab a spoonful of honey for a cough—often, it will work like magic. **Time spent:** 5 minutes to do a Web search for the closest bee farmer, 15 minutes (minus prep time) to make the cough medicine, and 30 seconds a day to take your "dose" of oxymel or straight honey

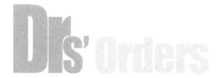

Drs' Orders
for Respiratory Health: Quit Smoking Now

Tobacco kills 5 million people every year worldwide, which is more than car accidents, suicide, AIDS, drugs, alcohol, and murder combined. According to the American Heart Association, over 45 million Americans are trapped by their addiction to smoking, and many are looking for a way to kick the habit before it mule-kicks them.

Cigarette smoking is the major cause of COPD and lung cancer. Smoking restricts your air passages and complicates your breathing. You endure chronic systemic inflammation, swelling in your lungs, and chronic bronchitis. Cigarette smoke kills lung cells and can trigger biological changes that mutate into cancer. Smoking affects your body in a number of ways, including causing respiratory problems and premature aging and increasing your risks of heart disease, vascular disease, stroke, and cancer. When you quit, you begin to reverse many of these health problems almost immediately.

We're not saying it's easy—not by any stretch. Try some of these suggestions from Dr. Linda Hyder Ferry, associate professor, Preventive Medicine and Family Medicine, Loma Linda University School of Medicine, and make this your first smoke-free year.

- Change your attitude. Tell yourself you can learn to live without tobacco. Focus on what you're getting (energy, freedom, better health, fewer colds) rather than on what you're giving up (the chance to die early, yay!). Instead of saying, "I'm quitting smoking," say, "I'm freeing myself from cigarettes."

- Get professional help. Talk to your doc about whether medications are right for you. One National Institutes of Health study found that when people used the nicotine patch for 24 weeks instead of the standard 8 weeks, it helped them stay smoke-free and made it easier for them to quit again if they had a slipup.

- Speak to a smoking cessation specialist, and maybe even join a support group at your local hospital. Find someone you can call when you have the urge to smoke, someone who can remind you of your goals and who can be supportive without being critical.

- Change your environment. Keep your home, car, and workplace smoke-free, and make sure you have something else to do in those places rather than smoke. If you need to hold something in your hand to take the place of a cigarette, you might want to try a cinnamon stick or a pen or pencil.

- If you need to simulate the feel of a cigarette in your mouth, drink ice-cold water through a straw. This will also stimulate chemicals in the brain that release dopamine, much as nicotine does.

- If you think every day doesn't count, consider this: Within 24 hours of smoking your last cigarette, your risk of having a major heart attack has decreased by 50 percent. It may not feel like you're making progress, but look at what you can accomplish in just 1 day! Once you are smoke-free, your body is going to look much better—your skin will be smoother and more radiant, your hair will soften and get shinier. And, of course, you'll smell better! You may have dulled your senses of taste and smell, but after you break free, you'll get back the enjoyment to be gotten from those senses, too.

If you need help to free yourself from cigarettes, you can call 800-QUIT-NOW (800-784-8669) or visit www.BecomeAnEx.org. Come to www.thedoctorstv.com and start a discussion thread to communicate with other people who are looking to break those chains. Don't just go it alone! We're in it with you!

Chapter Five

Go with Your Gut

We all have our own way of thinking about food. For some, food is fuel. For others, it's pleasure. For most, it's a combination of the two—but in any case, we tend to stop thinking about it the second the last bite goes down our throats.

The digestive tract may seem like merely a chute down which we pour pre-eaten food and remove, ahem, post-eaten food. Many people are surprised to find out that what happens in the middle is critical to the good health and even the survival of the entire body: A large part of our immune system is also located in the intestinal tract. The content of our diet has everything to do with our resistance to infection and disease, our energy level, our skin tone— even the speed at which our body ages. Eating habits that emphasize high-quality nutrition have a ripple effect that spreads through all the body systems.

Fix It in 5
Keep Your Digestion Running Smoothly

1. Drink plenty of water.
2. Eat a variety of fiber-rich foods, including whole grains and organic fruits and vegetables.
3. Take a walk every day.
4. Restock your digestive tract with "good" gut bacteria by eating fermented foods and taking probiotic supplements.
5. Avoid pathogens: Cook meat and eggs thoroughly, keep kitchen counters clean, and guard against food spoilage.

For millennia, our ancestors ate a steady diet that was highly nutritious for one simple reason: They didn't have a choice. Processed food hadn't been invented. So every meal was made from scratch with whole foods—there just weren't any other kinds.

Although canned foods came along in the 19th century and frozen foods in the early 20th

I know I'm supposed to eat fresh fruits and
vegetables, but the fact is, I'm too cheap. They're
expensive! Canned foods and meats like hot dogs
and hamburgers are just so much cheaper and easier.
Why is it so expensive to eat healthy?

Dr. Jim says . . .

I hear you. If I could wave a magic wand to get one thing, it would be to make organic fruits and vegetables cost next to nothing—and processed foods and sodas cost a fortune. Because, in a way, they
already do, but on the back end (yours!) and by making medical costs higher.

One thing is for sure—some outdated government policies sure are not helping the average family.
Take a look at this graphic from the Physicians Committee for Responsible Medicine that compares the
foods our federal government subsidizes with the foods our federal government recommends that we
eat. Notice anything odd?

The very foods that are undeniably linked to obesity, high blood pressure, diabetes, heart
disease—all the conditions that shorten our lives and increase health care costs—are all heavily
subsidized by tax dollars. Factory farms that produce meat and dairy products, grains, fats,
and sugars receive almost 98 percent of the federal subsidies. Yet the foods our bodies do best
with—legumes, nuts, vegetables, and fruits—receive a mere 2.3 percent. What's wrong with this
picture?

To trim your food costs, make fruits, vegetables, and organic meats and dairy products your top
food priorities. They may cost more now, but their long-term health benefits are priceless. With your
remaining food budget, shop discount big-box stores for staples like dried beans, oatmeal, jarred
tomato sauce, and whole wheat pasta.

If you have to cut corners on your grocery list, really question those "treats" for the kids—no one needs the cost or the constant temptation in the house. Not to mention, the word "treats" means "a special food that tastes good, especially one that you do not eat very often." They should not be a daily thing.

To help younger kids understand why you're limiting their treats, explain what excess sugar does to the body ("They taste good in your mouth, but your body says, 'Yuck!'"). Channel your teen's rebellious streak into a letter-writing protest campaign: Have him or her write your congressperson (go to www.house.gov/zip/ZIP2Rep.html and type in your zip code) to let him or her know that your family would like federal subsidies for farms to be in line with the stated nutritional objectives of this country.

Why Does a Salad Cost More Than a Big Mac?

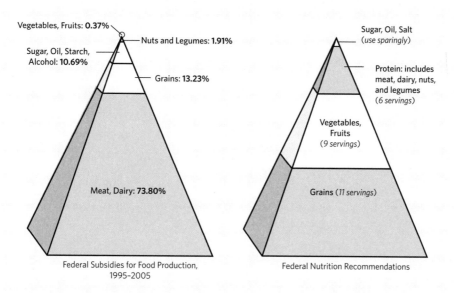

Vegetables, Fruits: **0.37%**
Nuts and Legumes: **1.91%**
Sugar, Oil, Starch, Alcohol: **10.69%**
Grains: **13.23%**
Meat, Dairy: **73.80%**

Federal Subsidies for Food Production, 1995–2005

Sugar, Oil, Salt (*use sparingly*)
Protein: includes meat, dairy, nuts, and legumes (*6 servings*)
Vegetables, Fruits (*9 servings*)
Grains (*11 servings*)

Federal Nutrition Recommendations

Source: Physicians committee for Responsible Medicine

century, it wasn't until World War II that the popularity of processed foods made a big leap in America and we became a culture hooked on convenience. During the 1950s, food chemists gave us everything from instant rice and processed cheese sauce to cake mixes and refrigerated cookie dough. No longer would Mom be chained to the stove!

But over the last 50 years, we've taken what was a liberating, time-saving novelty and made it into the mainstay of our diet. According to Eric Schlosser, author of *Fast Food Nation,* today, 90 percent of the average American family's food budget is spent on processed foods.

While we certainly have saved ourselves some time behind the stove, we're only just starting to uncover what that saved time has cost us in terms of health: The incidences of obesity, heart disease, cancer, and diabetes have all skyrocketed during those years. When combined with the other time-savers—escalators, drive-thrus, remote controls, microwave ovens—those processed foods that were once the ticket to freedom have now trapped many of us into carrying excess pounds and developing chronic diseases.

So what to do? This is one place where reversing just a few of those time-savers will pay tremendous health dividends. Yes, buying fresh vegetables and chopping them up might take more time than cranking open a can. True, until you get the hang of it, planning menus in advance seems like an annoying extra step when you could just pick up a frozen dinner and pop it in the microwave. But we have to change our mind-sets: Making healthy choices does not waste time, it creates it. And that's what we're interested in here, isn't it?

Our bodies get every single ounce of their energy from our food. And just as many of us would never dream of putting leaded gas into our shiny new cars, we need to take even a small amount of the same care with our bodies.

We know it's not easy—and in some ways, the deck is stacked against us. According to experts at Cornell University, since the late 1970s and early 1980s, the cost of fresh fruits and vegetables has increased by nearly 40 percent, while the price of soda has decreased by 25 percent. The hard truth is, there's money to be made selling those jars, cans, and boxes, and the processed food industry isn't going to give up our dollars without a fight. But, if we collectively commit to eating more of the old-school foods our ancestors ate before the 1950s

WHAT YOUR BODY'S TRYING TO TELL YOU: HEARTBURN AND GERD

When stomach acid splashes upward into your esophagus, your chest or throat feels like it's on fire—and you need relief. The tips below will soothe the pain of heartburn and gastro-esophageal reflux disease (GERD, which is a more serious problem that can damage your esophagus). See your doctor if heartburn persists for several weeks or if you think you have GERD. How can you tell? Heartburn is usually a pain behind your breastbone; you'll feel GERD at the back of your throat and may also cough and feel pain in your neck or face.

Skip your triggers. If you know you're at risk when you eat certain foods, by all means, avoid them. Common culprits include fizzy sodas, high-fat foods like pizza, acidic or spicy foods, coffee, and peppermint, as well as alcohol, nicotine, and caffeine. Studies show that different foods and beverages ignite heartburn pain for different people, so pay attention to what sets yours off.

Sleep like this. Don't let nighttime heartburn steal your sleep. Try waiting 3 hours to lie down after a meal. When you are in bed, sleep on your left side—that can cut your odds for heartburn in half (in contrast, sleeping on your right side relaxes the muscle that normally keeps gastric acids in your stomach). Get a wedge pillow, too. In one study published in the *Archives of Internal Medicine*, people who propped their heads up about 11 inches reduced their heartburn dramatically. And skip sleeping pills. Benzodiazepines such as diazepam, alpra-zolam, and triazolam doubled the risk for GERD in one study.

Start simply with drugs. Antacids (Maalox, Mylanta, Gelusil, Rolaids, and Tums) neutralize stomach acid. Look for a type containing alginates or alginic acid (such as Gaviscon-2 or Gena-ton) for the additional comfort of a protective coating deposited over the stomach contents so it can't backwash as easily. In one meta-analysis of over-the-counter GERD therapies published in the journal *Alimentary Pharmacy & Therapeutics*, researchers found that antacids containing algi-nates improved mild heartburn by 60 percent, compared to 11 percent for plain antacids.

Add an H2 blocker. For pain not relieved by antacids alone, try an over-the-counter H2 blocker such as cimetidine (Tagamet), famotidine (Pepcid), or ranitidine (Zantac). Take it a half hour before you eat a meal. These medications work by reducing the production of stomach acid and can ease symptoms about 70 percent of the time.

Ask your doctor about acid-stopping proton pump inhibitors. If you're still not feeling relief, step it up a bit. Available over the counter and by prescription, proton pump inhibitors block acid production in your stomach, stopping pain and allowing damaged tissue in your esophagus to heal. Take these for the shortest amount of time possible.

and we combine that with the technological advancements made in medicine over the past 50-plus years, there's no telling how long (and how well) we could live. We simply have no idea what that level of health would look like on a national scale.

This kind of change begins with us, each one of us, making a personal commitment to take care of our body and our family on a day-after-day, meal-after-meal basis. But first, let's talk about how the digestive system is built to wring every last nutrient out of our foods. Once you learn about it, it will be crystal clear that it's important to feed it well.

A 5-Minute Tour of Your Digestive System

Our bodies are the original waste management system: We break down the foods we eat into energy, and then we compost and eliminate the rest as waste. And while the entire culinary industry—cookbook publishers, foodies, food processors, farmer's markets, and the like— often goes to great lengths to create elaborate meals having multiple ingredients and varying colors and textures, our bodies still see food in these very clear-cut terms: energy and waste.

The act of digestion actually starts with the brain. When you see a piece of chocolate cake and inhale its delicious aroma, your brain signals the salivary glands to start producing saliva. You bite into the cake and some of your 5,000 to 10,000 taste buds, which live in the little bumps on your tongue called papillae, sort the flavors into the four basic tastes of sweet, salty, sour, and bitter and then send messages back up to the brain: "Yep, it's sweet, just like you thought." All that extra saliva helps moisten the food to make it easier to swallow, and the enzymes in the saliva start to break down some of the starches and sugars. Add to that the mashing your teeth do as you chew, and it's clear that digestion is well underway before you even swallow!

Keep Things Moving

Once you swallow, the cake travels down the esophagus and into the stomach. The cake makes it through the trapdoor at the base of the esophagus—the lower esophageal sphincter (unfortunate name, huh?)—and that valve closes to make sure the food doesn't go back up into the esophagus. Stomach enzymes and acids, working in conjunction with the stomach muscles to churn up the cake like a blender, pulverize the cake into a bunch of mush, called chyme, that can more easily pass into the intestine.

As the chocolate cake chyme (yummy!) travels through the small intestine to the large intestine, tiny projections on the walls of the small intestine suck up and absorb nutrients into the bloodstream. (Not that chocolate cake has much to offer nutrition-wise, but the process is the same whether you've eaten broccoli or bacon bits.) Once the chyme reaches the large intestine, there's really nothing left but water and waste. The large intestine removes the water so what's left can enter the colon as solid waste, and then exit as a sinker or a floater.

When everything is working perfectly, food goes in the mouth, gives up its nutrients as it travels through the body, and exits the body as waste, and you can ignore it because you don't feel a thing. But unfortunately, when things go wrong in the digestive process, eating can cause discomfort or even pain. For example, if that valve in your lower esophagus doesn't work properly due to gastroesophageal reflux disease (GERD) or esophagitis, your stomach contents may gurgle back up into the esophagus and cause burning and discomfort after you eat.

If food moves through the intestines too quickly, there isn't enough time to get all of the water out and you may experience diarrhea. If it moves too slowly, too much water is removed and the waste has trouble getting through the colon—and you could get constipated. No fun.

While the body is capable of digesting all types of foods, certain foods glide through the digestive tract more easily while others are more cumbersome, which can strain or damage the colon. High-fiber foods are eliminated more easily because they tend to have a nice balance between water and bulk, while foods low in fiber linger longer in the intestines, leading to constipation and hemorrhoids. When fiber gets to the colon, the normal bacteria living there ferment it to support their growth and repopulate the gut with more of their own kind of healthful bacteria. This is the so-called prebiotic effect: when we eat certain foods, we enhance the strength and numbers of the beneficial bacteria in our bellies.

Ultimately, most issues with clearing out the innards can be solved with those two magic words: fiber and water. Fruits and vegetables have both!

Have a Blast

When you first adopt a higher-fiber diet, you may encounter greater amounts of a necessary evil in the digestive process: gas.

Everyone has gas. According to the National Institute of Diabetes and Digestive and Kidney Diseases, it's totally normal to pass gas about 14 times a day—truly—and to produce somewhere between 1 and 4 pints of gas every day. (Knowing that makes you feel a little better, doesn't it?)

Some gas can arise simply because of swallowing air while eating quickly, drinking through a straw, chewing gum, or drinking carbonated soda—but most of that gas quickly retreats as burps. But the gas that retreats through the other end is a natural result of the breakdown of foods by the "good" bacteria that live harmlessly in our colons. These bacteria help digest food that could not be processed by the stomach or small intestine. However, in this process, hydrogen, carbon dioxide, and, sometimes, stinky methane are produced, and they exit the body just like waste—often causing our loved ones to exit the room at the same time.

For every 10 grams (2 teaspoons) of fiber that you eat, your intestinal bacteria produce, on average, a quart of gas as a by-product of fermentation. That's why eating fiber can cause a little extra flatulence, bloating, or belly bulge. If you are adding fiber to your diet, start with a small amount (about 3 to 5 grams a day) and build up the dose gradually.

Everyone has a different balance of bacteria in their intestines, and therefore some people experience more gas than others. Likewise, some people's bodies produce methane and some don't, which is why not everyone has Uncle Charlie's level of stinky gas. Although it is usually

I want to eat more beans, but how
do I avoid the smelly side effects?

Dr. Travis says . . .

High in fiber, rich in health-protecting antioxidants, and loaded with protein, beans just may be the perfect food, except for one infamous little glitch—the gassy aftereffects. Fortunately, you can enjoy beans without embarrassment. Here's how.

Start with small portions. Beans contain large amounts of raffinose, a complex sugar your body can't easily break down. The job of doing so goes to beneficial bacteria in your digestive system that produce smelly hydrogen sulfide and other gases as they work. Starting with very small helpings of beans and working up to regular-size portions (such as a starter portion of $\frac{1}{4}$ cup of beans on a salad or a modest $\frac{1}{2}$ cup of chili as a main dish) minimizes this stinky side effect.

Pack some Beano. Sprinkling a few drops of this gas-stopping product on your first forkful of beans can significantly reduce the gas you produce after a meal, researchers say. Beano contains an enzyme that breaks down the sugars in beans. (Other products with alpha-galactosidase enzyme may also have the same effect.)

Rinse often. You can reduce the raffinose in beans by rinsing canned beans thoroughly. If you start with dried beans, be sure to rinse them after soaking and again after cooking the beans (before you add them to the dish you're making).

Add a gas-reducing spice. Seasoning bean dishes with garlic and ginger (either fresh or dried) during cooking can reduce the gas they produce. The herb epazote, also known as Mexican tea (and often used in Mexican cooking), may help, too.

harmless, gas can cause discomfort when it fills up the colon and presses on the abdomen—which is why you're not alone in thinking that farting feels good. (If you feel the need in public, don't make yourself miserable. It's natural, so why fight it? Just excuse yourself, hit the toilet and let 'er rip.)

For most of us, embarrassing levels of gas don't happen that often, and if they do, they're usually brought on by a greasy lunch or a broccoli binge. But some people struggle with ongoing cases of serious gas. One of the least understood causes of this is irritable bowel syndrome (IBS), a collection of symptoms with an unknown cause. People who suffer IBS may have trouble digesting certain foods, resulting in pain, cramping, gas, diarrhea, and constipation. While it's difficult to pinpoint the foods that bring IBS on, some have found that it may be triggered by certain foods (like chocolate or alcohol), stress, hormones, or gastroenteritis.

Clean It Up!

Since the establishment of the Food and Drug Administration in 1937, we've made great strides in food safety—but this country still has 76 million cases of food-related illness each year, according to the CDC. Because of the globalization of the food supply and the overuse of antibiotics and other drugs in humans and in our agricultural practices, certain antibiotic-resistant bacterial "superbugs" and other pathogens are continuing to gather strength. We overuse antibiotics, so resistant bugs colonize our bodies. In addition, livestock raised on factory farms are routinely given low doses of antibiotics to promote growth and prevent infections caused by overcrowding and unhygienic conditions. The bacteria that survive the antibiotics are the strongest of their colonies, and they pass their heightened resistance to their offspring—which then propagate like mad and eventually end up on our plates—most of them killed by cooking, but many not.

Methicillin-resistant *Staphylococcus aureus,* or MRSA, is just one of the pathogens that have found their way into the food supply. *Helicobacter pylori,* the bug responsible for most stomach ulcers, spreads through food and water. In a study published in the *Journal of Food Safety,* a random sampling of poultry in a grocery store turned up nearly 40 percent of chicken testing positive for it. *Salmonella* strains routinely show up in national recalls of everything from peanut butter to dog food to ground meat. And here's the biggest bummer: Our first line of attack against most of these intestinal bad guys has been antibiotics.

But you know that adage "What doesn't kill you makes you stronger"?

Yes. We haven't killed them; we've made them stronger. And many are completely immune to our big guns now.

Luckily, there are some very simple ways to proactively protect ourselves from foodborne illnesses. Here are a few 5-minute health fixes that can strengthen our defenses so we can ward off bugs before they take hold—and help us fight if they've already gotten in.

WHAT YOUR BODY'S TRYING TO TELL YOU: ABDOMINAL PAIN

Pain in your belly can be tough to diagnose at home. Sometimes it's simple indigestion. Other times, it may be a signal that you need prompt medical attention. Here's how to tell the difference. (And of course, call your doctor or 911 if you think your pain is a medical emergency.)

Symptoms: Discomfort, bloating, pain in your upper abdomen. May be relieved by belching or even throwing up.
What it could mean: Possibly just indigestion from a large meal, a new medication, stress, too much caffeine or other acidic foods or drinks
What to do: Cut back on indigestion triggers. If discomfort persists for more than 2 weeks, is severe, or if you have any other troubling symptoms, call your doctor.

Symptoms: Sharp pain in lower right abdomen, sometimes with nausea, vomiting, and/or fever.
What it could mean: Appendicitis
What to do: Call 911 or go to the emergency room immediately.

Symptoms: Pain in upper right abdomen, it may spread to your right shoulder, chest, or back; sometimes with nausea, vomiting, or intestinal gas.
What it could mean: Gallstones
What to do: Call your doctor.

Symptoms: A burning pain in the chest, sometimes with a sour taste in your mouth and/or trouble swallowing.
What it could mean: Heartburn or gastroesophageal reflux disease (GERD)
What to do: Take an antacid or try an acid-blocking heartburn medicine from the drugstore. See your doctor if pain persists.

Symptom: For women, sharp pain or ache on one side of the lower abdomen at the mid-point of your menstrual cycle.
What it could mean: "Mittelschmerz"—the medical term for pain when an egg is released from one of your ovaries at ovulation
What to do: Usually, you don't have to do anything about this normal ache. An over-the-counter pain reliever like ibuprofen can help, though. See your doctor if the pain is extremely severe, seems to change, or if you also have vaginal bleeding at mid-cycle.

Symptoms: Sharp, cramping, or even a dull pain in the upper abdomen; it may come and go, and may spread to your back below your right shoulder blade. May happen soon after eating or several hours after having several alcoholic drinks.

What it could mean: Pancreatitis

What to do: Call 911 or go to the emergency room immediately.

Symptoms: A bloated feeling and/or pain or pressure in the abdomen with fewer than three bowel movements a week. Stools may be hard, dry, and difficult to pass.

What it could mean: Constipation

What to do: Start by increasing the fiber and fluids in your diet; daily exercise may help, too. If constipation doesn't clear up, see your doctor.

Symptoms: Bloating or a dull ache after having milk, ice cream, or other dairy products.

What it could mean: Lactose intolerance

What to do: Skip dairy products or use products that help digest lactose in them. If you stop eating dairy products, consider taking a calcium supplement to protect your bones.

Symptoms: Cramping pains throughout your abdomen, with bloating, fatigue, gas, constipation, and/or diarrhea.

What it could mean: Irritable bowel syndrome

What to do: Stress reduction and a lower-fat diet can help. Slowly increasing the fiber in your diet may relieve constipation. See your doctor if problems continue.

Symptoms: A gnawing stomach pain that eases up after you eat and returns when your stomach is empty. Sometimes with indigestion, heartburn, nausea.

What it could mean: A peptic ulcer or gastritis—inflammation of the stomach lining

What to do: Call 911 or go to the emergency room if you have signs of a bleeding ulcer—throwing up blood or something that looks like coffee grounds, black or bloody stools, feeling faint and chilly. Otherwise, you can take an antacid or acetaminophen for pain. Call your doctor for an evaluation and treatment.

Symptoms: Stubborn pain, with yellowing of the skin and whites of the eyes and dark urine.

What it could mean: Viral hepatitis

What to do: Call the doctor immediately.

Symptoms: Back pain that spreads to include the rib cage and groin area.

What it could mean: Kidney stones

What to do: Call the doctor immediately.

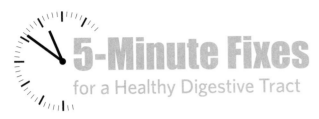

5-Minute Fixes
for a Healthy Digestive Tract

By basing our diets on plant-based foods—vegetables, fruits, whole grains, legumes, nuts, and seeds—and then adding lean protein (deepwater fish and organic lean meats, eggs, and low-fat dairy products), and using monounsaturated fats like olive oil and canola oil, we can create a solid foundation of health that can help us prevent (and sometimes reverse!) nearly every chronic disease on the planet and give ourselves the best chance of withstanding a superbug infection. (Notice that we did not include sugar in our list of health-promoting foods—with good reason!)

A nutrient-dense diet—one that packs the maximum nutrition into the minimum number of calories—is the ultimate time-creator. It will give your body the most energy for living life to the fullest now as well as the nourishment it needs to protect your body systems over the long term. The beauty of many digestive system health fixes is how simple they are: You can start to make positive changes with the very next bite you put in your mouth.

Sprinkle cayenne pepper on every dish you can. Those *H. pylori* bugs that cause sores called ulcers in the lining of the stomach are actually everywhere—one of every two human stomachs in the world, according to the NIH. Not everyone who has them will develop ulcers, and most people don't even know the bacteria are there. But these little critters can get into our bodies when we're babies and stick to our stomach walls for decades, drawing nutrients from our food and hiding behind the layer of mucus that protects the stomach. While antibiotic treatment may work in theory, all too often the *H. pylori* live on in there.

Based on research from the *Critical Review of Food Science Nutrition,* one of the best ways to prevent ulcers caused by *H. pylori* may be the opposite of what you might suspect: Eating chile

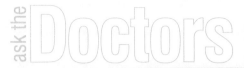

ask the Doctors

Can you give me one good reason other than my weight that I should eat more fiber?

Here are several! The zero-calorie insoluble fiber that fills you up and cuts your cravings also ensures that your digestion will hum along nicely. Soluble fiber—the type in apples, kidney beans, and oat bran—forms a gel in your digestive tract that helps prevent your intestines from absorbing cholesterol. Fiber can even help you manage your blood sugar. Aim high: A *New England Journal of Medicine* study found that 50 grams of fiber a day helped people with diabetes manage their blood sugar by slowing their body's absorption of carbohydrates. A few delicious ways to get to 50 grams:

Almonds: Twenty-three almonds (a good handful) net you 3.5 grams of fiber and 6 grams of satisfying protein. Have slivered almonds in salads, raw almonds for a snack, chopped almonds in chicken salad, or even crushed almonds as a coating for baked chicken breasts.

Oatmeal: A special fiber—beta glucan—in oats has been proven, in a study in the *American Journal of Therapeutics,* to lower LDL cholesterol by up to 30 percent in people with high cholesterol. Up the fiber of a serving even more by adding fresh berries.

Apples: Leave the skins on (for pears and sweet potatoes, too) and net 2.3 grams of soluble fiber for each. A Brazilian study found that women could lower their blood sugar, triglycerides, and total cholesterol just by adding three apples or pears a day to a weight-management plan.

Supplements: Drink a glass of fiber supplement made from psyllium that has 2.4 grams of soluble fiber per serving before a meal for even better calorie control and blood sugar balance.

*—**Mitzi Dulan, RD,** nutritionist*
and coauthor of The All-Pro Diet

peppers! Capsaicin, the active ingredient in chile peppers, actually kills bacteria as they arrive in the gut while also stimulating the stomach lining to generate more protective secretions and mucus. As a bonus, cayenne also stimulates blood flow—people from cultures that use a lot of chile peppers in their cooking tend to have the lowest rates of heart disease and high blood pressure. (We love it when these fixes have multiple benefits!)

If you like the flavor and don't mind spicy food, you might try eating cayenne as often as possible. (If you already have an ulcer, you may want to be a bit cautious—spicy foods may exacerbate your condition.) Consider going to restaurants serving foods from cultures that use a lot of chili powder, such as Thai and Mexican, and ask for your dish to be made as spicy as you can handle it. Add Tabasco to chili, bean soups, jambalaya. Sprinkle chili powder over popcorn. If you can stand the heat, those bugs won't stand a chance. **Time spent:** 20 seconds to sprinkle chili powder or hot sauce on food

Take a probiotic capsule daily. Years of antibacterial overuse—in everything from soaps to toothpastes—have left our "good" gut bacteria severely compromised. But a thriving population of these bacteria helps not only our digestion, but our overall immunity as well. By reinforcing these strong gut soldiers, called probiotics, we strengthen from the inside our defenses against bad bugs, yeast, and other intestinal infections.

Many delicious foods have high levels of these beneficial bacteria, including yogurt, miso, and fermented and unfermented milk. Unfortunately, many of these foods are an acquired taste, and if you don't appreciate that sour tang, you might not get their health benefits. If that's the case with you, or if you would like the quickest way to pump up the populations of "good" bacteria in your belly, you can take probiotic capsules. Available in the refrigerated sections of your health food store, high-quality probiotic supplements offer a dose of anywhere from 50 million colony-forming units (CFUs) per day to more than 1 trillion CFUs per day. A recent meta-analysis of 31 randomized, placebo-controlled studies, published in the *World Journal of Gastroenterology,* found the probiotic *S. boulardii* could be "strongly recommended for the prevention of antibiotic-associated diarrhea and traveler's diarrhea." Plenty of other promising research suggests that probiotics can:

I love spicy foods, but why do they make
it hurt so much when I go number two?

Dr. Lisa says . . .

When you eat spicy foods, the spices actually maintain their structure after you eat them, so as they travel all the way through your digestive tract, they retain their "heat," possibly irritating the lining of the digestive tract and causing diarrhea in some people. Just as they do when they touch your mouth, when those ingredients touch your anus, it burns. Contrary to many people's beliefs, spicy foods don't cause hemorrhoids or ulcers, but they may exacerbate those conditions. Mix in foods like rice or sugar to dilute the spice.

- Keep harmful pathogens from implanting in the intestinal wall
- Improve the function of the mucous lining of the intestinal tract
- Help manage symptoms of IBS
- Help you recover from intestinal, vaginal, and urinary tract infections
- Enhance immunity and decrease systemic inflammation
- Help prevent or reduce the severity of colds and flu
- Possibly even help prevent cavities!

When we consider the research that suggests probiotics may also help reduce the recurrence of bladder cancer, there's no doubt—many doctors are pro probiotics! **Time spent:** 5 minutes picking out a bottle at the store; 20 seconds a day taking your dose

Count the ingredients. If there are more than five ingredients, eat the food rarely. If the ingredient list has more than 20 items, take a pass or just throw the food away. You don't need to eat any food with an ingredient list that looks like a vocabulary quiz for a chemical engineer. As our pal Jillian Michaels, trainer and life coach on NBC's *The Biggest Loser,* likes to say, "Only eat things that come from the ground or have a mother." This edict will steer you toward fresh, whole foods and away from the processed foods that add way too much sodium, hydrogenated fat, and chemical additives and preservatives to your diet. **Time spent:** 5 minutes in each aisle of the grocery store, taking your time to choose wisely (or, better yet, shop the outer walls!)

Check the label on your hot dogs—especially before you grill. As we become more aware of the risks of certain additives and preservatives in our food, a few stand out as absolute no-brainers to avoid, such as sodium nitrate and sodium nitrite. Often used in processed meats to preserve their pink color and "smoky" flavor, these preservatives have been shown to increase the incidence of colorectal cancers. Those risks can be amplified by the formation of hydrocarbons, substances found in meat when it is cooked at high temperatures over an open flame. Indeed, a study from the University of South Carolina in Columbia found that the women who ate the most grilled, barbecued, or smoked red meat over their lifetimes had a 47 percent increased risk of breast cancer compared to those who ate the least. If they didn't eat very many fruits and vegetables, their increased risk jumped to 74 percent.

With the tremendous variety of foods available today, you no longer have to give up hot dogs to give up nitrates! Many brands offer "uncured" meats that use natural curing agents rather than excessive salt and additives. And if you like the taste of grilled meat, you can minimize your exposure to hydrocarbons by sticking to lean meats that don't drip juices on the flame—the resulting smoke that floats up and engulfs the meat is the source of the problem. **Time spent:** 5 extra minutes to read labels in the store the first time; zero extra time to remove hot dogs from the grill before smoke can develop

Order a seltzer maker. We've all heard the bad news about soda. At this stage, we should really be calling it "liquid cigarettes." (Or, as it's referred to in Dr. Jim's office, "diabetes in a bottle.") Consider:

- Over the last decade, according to the American Heart Association, consumption of soda and sugar-sweetened beverages has contributed to 130,000 new cases of diabetes and 14,000 new cases of coronary heart disease.

- One 12-ounce soda has approximately 150 calories and 40 grams of sugar in the form of high-fructose corn syrup, which is equal to approximately 10 teaspoons of sugar.

Doctors

My family has a history of cancer, and
I'm very interested in doing everything
I can to prevent it. What are the three
most important things for me to do?

These are my top three suggestions:

1. Pay attention to the food you eat: Avoid industrial foods and sugar and make sure to eat what I call "Anticancer" vegetables and fruits (such as extra virgin olive oil, berries, stone fruits, fish, organic meat, omega-3 eggs, lentils, beans, cruciferous vegetables, tomatoes, whole grains and more). Also, drink green tea every day, and add turmeric powder to your meals three times a week.

2. Walk or jog or dance or move your body in whatever other way you enjoy at least 30 minutes five to six times a week.

3. Avoid the most common sources of pollution around you to the extent possible: tobacco smoke, pesticides (especially in your house and garden), dry cleaning chemicals, phthalates and parabens of many perfumes and cosmetics, BPA of hard plastics (especially from heating food or liquids in plastic containers in a microwave).

*—**David Servan-Schreiber, MD, PhD,** cofounder of the Center for Integrative Medicine at the University of Pittsburgh Medical Center and author of the international bestseller* Anticancer, *translated into 36 languages worldwide*

- According to findings from the National Health and Nutrition Examination Survey (NHANES 1999–2004), two or more sugary sodas a day may increase the risk of early kidney damage by 86 percent.

- Soda contains phosphoric acid, which weakens bones by leaching calcium from them and erodes the enamel on teeth.

- Soda can actually unclog a drain—imagine what it's doing to your insides!

One

Drink, 14 Benefits
Water

Over the course of an average Starbucks–Diet Coke–Bud Light day, the one drink our bodies really need can be forgotten: water. Water is the most essential element for life, and it is vital for every cellular function. The human body is composed of 60 to 70 percent water—the average 160-pound female is made up of approximately 14 gallons of water!

But people who drink less than two glasses (16 ounces) of water a day are considered chronically dehydrated, and their risk for heart attack is double that of people who drink more than five glasses (40 ounces). Their hearts can enlarge to two times the normal size and beat twice as fast as healthy, hydrated hearts. When you don't take in enough water, your blood becomes very thick—and the thicker, or more viscous, blood is, the harder it is for it to circulate normally, taxing the entire circulatory system. You also feel groggy, dizzy, and tired—and are likely to get a headache.

Water should be your first go-to beverage when you're thirsty—and even before you are. Aim for at least six to eight glasses of water a day, and more if you are exercising or are experiencing a summer heat wave. Check out all the ways that water helps us function at our best:

And lest you think this pertains only to sugar-sweetened cola, think again: Diet soda may be no better. In addition to retaining sugary sodas' phosphoric acid bone-compromising effect, it might also compromise your kidneys. One Harvard study, presented at the American Society of Nephrology's 42nd Annual Meeting and Scientific Exposition, analyzed research on 3,200 women who drank two or more servings of artificially sweetened soda per day and found that they had a 30 percent drop in their kidney function—an effect not seen in those who drank sugar-sweetened soda.

If the thought of giving up your sparkly beverage strikes fear in your heart, please know you don't have to. In fact, your regular glass of soda could be a time-creator. A household seltzer maker allows you to increase your fluid intake by using your own filtered water to make clean, cold,

1. Keeps the belly full and satiated
2. Increases the metabolic rate (bonus: drinking two glasses of cold water could burn an extra 50 calories)
3. Lowers blood pressure
4. Enhances skin tone
5. Improves immunity
6. Prevents some types of headaches
7. Helps flush out toxins released during fat burning
8. Regulates body temperature
9. Carries nutrients and oxygen to all cells in the body
10. Protects and cushions vital organs and joints
11. Aids in the conversion of food to energy
12. Provides a vehicle for removing waste from the body
13. Makes possible the tremendous increase in blood flow required during pregnancy
14. Helps the brain to focus and concentrate

To make water more appealing, try sweetening it naturally: Fill your glass of H_2O with mint leaves or with slices of oranges, lemons, limes, strawberries, peaches, cucumber, or ginger. Use a pitcher water filter such as those made by Brita and keep the pitcher in the fridge, or invest in a fridge with a filtered water dispenser. Get a stainless steel bottle and fill it up with fresh, cold water to take with you every time you leave the house. (Bonus: You won't be contributing to the 2.5 million plastic bottles that, according to the Clean Air Council, are used every hour in America.)

sparkling, natural sodas anytime you'd like. After an initial investment of $80 to $100 (visit www.sodaclub.com), you'll enjoy years of homemade seltzer for pennies per bottle—and no wasteful disposable containers overflowing in your recycling bin! Squeeze in a lemon, pour in a splash of OJ or cranberry juice, or even—if you just can't live without it—get some organic cola-flavored syrup (www.naturesflavors.com). Even if you are a complete soda addict, you don't have to subject your body to high-fructose corn syrup or artificial sweeteners ever again. **Time spent:** 5 minutes ordering a seltzer maker online, 3 minutes to set it up, and 60 seconds to create your own bottle of soda

Choose an organic apple. And grab some organic grapes. Why? Think back to our discussion about food at the beginning of the chapter. Our bodies had a good thing going there for a while. We fed them the fresh foods that we'd planted and tended or stalked and killed with our own hands. Once we domesticated animals, we likely ate a chicken within a few hours of slaughtering it. We ate only seasonal produce; there was no freighter to haul strawberries up from Latin America during the winter. We had only what we could scrounge up or can or otherwise preserve ahead of time.

That's not the way it works today. In fact, today, we are as far removed from the process of raising our own food as we've ever been.

According to the President's Cancer Panel, of the more than 80,000 to 100,000 synthetic chemicals currently being used in our environment, only 2 percent have been tested for their effects on human health. Our bodies are not meant to run on hydrogenated oils; high-fructose corn syrup; grains stripped of all their nutrition; animals force-fed antibiotics; or foods drenched in pesticides, herbicides, and other poisons. And, luckily, they don't have to. Simply by choosing organic foods, we can avoid almost all of those questionable chemicals and practices.

The Environmental Working Group (EWP) did a survey of produce and found what they call the Dirty Dozen—12 foods that, due to the high levels of toxic pesticide residue left on or in them when they're raised conventionally, you absolutely should buy organic. That applies to any fruit or vegetable that has a skin that you eat. The EWP estimates that by choosing organic when buying the following fruits and vegetables, you can reduce the amount of pesticides you ingest in your diet by 80 percent.

"THE DIRTY DOZEN"

- celery
- peaches
- strawberries
- apples
- blueberries
- nectarines
- bell peppers
- spinach

- kale
- cherries
- potatoes
- grapes (imported)

The EWP also found the fruits and vegetables that have the lowest detectible traces of pesticides; they aren't as dangerous when they've been raised conventionally. In general, fruits and vegetables with thick skins are usually safer because the pesticides cannot penetrate as readily to the edible part inside.

"THE CLEAN FIFTEEN"

- onions
- avocados
- sweet corn
- pineapple
- mangos
- sweet peas
- asparagus
- kiwi
- cabbage
- eggplant
- cantaloupe
- watermelon
- grapefruit
- sweet potatoes
- honeydew melon

The switch to organic is all the more important with little ones in the house: A recent study in *Pediatrics* found that children 8 to 15 years old with the highest level of pesticides in their blood also had the highest incidence of ADHD. For this and many other reasons, when possible, choose the organic apple over the conventional one. And the organic grapes, bell peppers, and carrots. And keep making those choices, on a minute-by-minute, food-by-food basis—ideally, with food grown right in your community. **Time spent:** 1 minute to choose organic over conventional produce in the grocery store and 1 fun and invigorating hour a week to shop at your local farmer's market (check out Local Harvest for the farmer's market near you: www.localharvest.org)

Drink 1 cup of green tea before or after lunch. A recent unpublished study from Taiwan found that drinking just 1 cup of green tea a day could drastically reduce your risk of lung cancer. In study participants who didn't smoke, the protective effect was more than fivefold; in smokers, the effect more than doubled, conferring a twelvefold decreased chance of lung cancer. Other studies have found that the more green tea people drink, the lower their risks are of developing many different kinds of cancer, including stomach, prostate, colorectal, esophageal, and pancreatic cancers. According to the NIH, still more research suggests that green tea may help control weight and may lower the risk of heart disease.

So, green tea is a multitasking time-creator, possibly helping you manage your weight as you profit from all of its tremendous health benefits. Buy organic green tea and savor a cup before or after a meal (preferably lunch, since green tea's caffeine may interfere with your sleep if you wait until dinnertime). If you drink it before your meal, you're more likely to eat slowly and, therefore, to eat less. If you drink it after the meal, you signal to your stomach, "That's it! Eating's done," and you'll be less likely to reach for seconds. **Time spent:** 5 minutes boiling the water and brewing a cup

Pack lunch with your teen. One recent study published in the journal *Preventing Chronic Disease* did an analysis of teens' lunch behavior. Those who brought their lunches from home 5 days a week ate less fast food, drank less soda, ate french fries and high-sugar foods less often, and ate more fruits and vegetables than their classmates who never brought lunch to school. Help your kid get a great start—for every extra year you can prevent adolescent

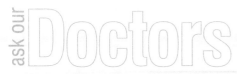

I don't drink to excess all the time—maybe once or twice a year, at most—but I always suffer mightily the next day. I wonder, is there any way to prevent a hangover?

Dr. Travis says . . .

While I would always caution you not to drink to excess, yes, there are ways you can help prevent a hangover. For example, drinking light-colored alcohol may reduce hangover symptoms. Research suggests that darker liquors such as whiskey and rum cause worse hangovers than lighter liquors such as vodka and gin. Congeners, toxic by-products of the fermentation process, are found in higher concentrations in darker liquors and contribute to more morning-after regret.

Make sure you pair each drink with water. For every glass of wine, ask for a glass of water. Consciously rehydrating like that will not only help prevent an awful hangover the next day, you'll also bolster your body's ability to protect itself from any free-floating germs and bugs out there, because drinking suppresses your immune system (a big reason to avoid drinking when you're sick). Drink responsibly and in moderation, and you won't have to worry about feeling so crappy the next day.

weight gain, a child's chances of avoiding adult obesity and related health problems—diabetes, heart disease, and so on—go down. While you're at it—pack your own! You don't need to spend the time or the calories on the deli or the company cafeteria. Invest in a cooler bag and some reusable glass containers with plastic tops. You might also bring baby carrots, grape tomatoes, chickpeas, and chopped cucumber to snack on during the day. Shoot to get half of your daily veggies by lunch, and you'll have serious healthy eating already in the bank by the time dinner rolls around. **Time spent:** 5 minutes every morning packing lunch and snacks

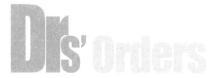

Drs' Orders

for Digestive Health and Enhanced Immunity:
Eat More Vegetables

We talked earlier in the chapter about nutrient-dense foods. Our goal should always be to fill our diets with as many high-quality, highly nutritious foods as possible. That, of course, starts with vegetables.

Vegetables are the one food group that really has no downside. Fruits have some (albeit natural) sugar; whole grains, when eaten in large quantities, can add up to extra calories. Even organic meat and dairy, though vastly better than hormone- and antibiotic-pumped conventional products, can have extra fat, too.

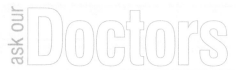

Is it bad that I only go poop a few times a week?

Some people are concerned if they don't have a bowel movement every day. Not to worry: Normal bowel movement frequency ranges from three times a week to twice a day, depending on your diet and your habit. There is no risk of being poisoned by poop if you do not have a daily bowel movement, so extraordinary measures need not be taken if you miss having one for a day or two. Your stools may become firmer and more difficult to pass, though.

—**Lawrence R. Schiller, MD,** *gastroenterologist*
at the Baylor Health Care System in Dallas, Texas

In contrast, vegetables are solidly in the "pro" column. Because of their high fiber and water content, which help smooth the way through the digestive system, they fill us up for very few calories, and even provide that satisfying *crunch!* when we need it. But perhaps most importantly, every single vegetable has a slightly different nutritional profile. Each one has its own formula—a combination of antioxidants, vitamins, and minerals that's different from all the others'. And we should look to the rainbow of those vegetables to draw the greatest benefit from our diets.

Throughout your day, aim to eat vegetables in as many colors of the rainbow as possible:

Green: Dark green leafy vegetables such as spinach and Swiss chard have omega-3 fatty acids and fiber; they lower cholesterol and decrease blood clotting. Other green vegetables and fruits include: arugula, asparagus, avocados, broccoli, green cabbage, honeydew melon, leeks, sugar snap peas, and zucchini.

Blue and purple: Eggplant is high in fiber and chlorogenic acid, which may help fight cancer and lower LDL cholesterol (according to lab research). Other blue and purple vegetables include: purple potatoes, asparagus, and cabbage.

Yellow and orange: Sweet potatoes are high in vitamin A, which is good for the eyes and bones. Other orange vegetables include: butternut squash, carrots, pumpkin, yellow bell peppers, and sweet corn.

Red: Tomatoes are a versatile nutritional multitasker, packed with antioxidants, vitamin C, fiber, and lycopene, one of the best-studied cancer fighters on the planet. Other red vegetables include: red onions, red bell peppers, rhubarb, and radicchio.

White: Cauliflower is incredibly high in vitamin C—you get 60 to 70 percent of your recommended daily allowance in 1 cup! Other white vegetables include: jicama, kohlrabi, mushrooms, onions, parsnips, and potatoes.

WHAT YOUR BODY'S TRYING TO TELL YOU: TOILET BOWL CLUES

Oddly colored urine. Strange-smelling bowel movements. Was it something you ate? Or does it reflect a deeper health problem? Here's how to tell.

READING YOUR STOOL

Symptoms: Light, white, or clay-colored bowel movement
What it could mean: Can be caused by taking diarrhea drugs containing bismuth subsalicylate (such as Kaopectate or Pepto-Bismol), or may be a sign of a problem in the system that drains the gallbladder, liver, and pancreas
What to do: Call your doctor.

Symptoms: Yellowish stool that may look greasy or have a very bad odor
What it could mean: May be a sign of an absorption disorder, such as celiac disease
What to do: See your doctor for an evaluation.

Symptoms: Black stool
What it could mean: Could be from iron supplements, diarrhea medications, black licorice, or even blueberries. May also be caused by bleeding in the upper intestinal tract, from an intestinal infection, inflammatory bowel disease, or bleeding from hemorrhoids.
What to do: Call your doctor right away.

Symptoms: Red stool
What it could mean: May be due to red food coloring, tomato products, beets, or cranberries, or may be a sign of bleeding in the lower intestinal tract
What to do: Call your doctor right away if you suspect bleeding is the cause.

Symptoms: Frequent loose, watery bowel movements (several times a day)
What it could mean: Diarrhea from a bacterial or viral infection
What to do: Drink plenty of fluids; if the diarrhea is severe or lasts for more than a few days, sip an electrolyte beverage (also called a rehydration drink) such as Pedialyte, CeraLyte, or Infalyte or a sports drink. See your doctor if the diarrhea gets worse, if you don't get better within 5 days (2 days for babies and children), if you have a fever above 101°F (100.4°F for children), or if there is blood or pus in your stool.

Symptoms: Green stool

What it could mean: Usually a reflection of what you've eaten, such as lots of green, leafy vegetables, green drinks or frozen pops, even iron supplements

What to do: Follow the advice given for diarrhea.

Symptoms: Small, hard, dry stools that may even be little balls (like deer or rabbit poop!)

What it could mean: Constipation

What to do: Increase the amount of fiber in your diet, drink more water, and get some exercise.

Symptoms: Lots of mucus on a regular basis, sometimes with blood

What it could mean: Crohn's disease or ulcerative colitis

What to do: See your doctor.

Symptoms: Stool that sinks or floats

What it could mean: It's a mostly harmless indicator of how much gas is in your stool. But if your stool sinks and is hard and dry, you may be constipated.

What to do: Usually, sinkers and floaters are nothing to worry about, and, in fact, experts are divided over which type is healthiest. Just be sure you're eating plenty of fiber-rich produce and whole grains and drinking six to eight glasses of water a day for easy "passage" of your bowel movements.

Symptoms: Soft (but not liquid), S-shaped bowel movement

What it could mean: A normal bowel movement

What to do: Keep on doing whatever you've been doing—a bowel movement like this is a good sign that you're getting plenty of fiber and water.

READING YOUR URINE

Symptoms: Cloudy urine (not translucent)

What it could mean: A urinary tract infection

What to do: Call your doctor.

Symptoms: Pink, red, or brown urine

What it could mean: Coloring from a medication you're taking or from foods like beets or blackberries. Could also be a sign of a liver disorder or bleeding in the urinary tract.

What to do: Call your doctor.

Each and every vegetable is a miraculous source of nature's medicine. And, when you choose organic over conventional produce, you get an added bonus: Rather than depending on pesticides to fight pests for them, organic vegetables fend off attacks with an arsenal of weapons called secondary plant metabolites, or SPMs. These natural chemicals are what give fruits and vegetables their amazing array of colors and flavors. When we eat them, the fruits and veggies pass along to our immune system the strength they've earned in the form of greater nutritional value and higher concentrations of antioxidants.

Do every single thing you can to add more vegetables to your life. Here are some measures you might want to try:

- Order pizzas with double the sauce and half of the cheese, and load on the veggies.

- Have a cup of vegetarian chili or bean soup as an appetite-quenching appetizer.

- Put carrots, celery, cucumber, grape tomatoes, radishes, and other crunchy crudités on the table for munching on before dinner is ready.

- Buy a juicer or high-quality blender and put a cup of spinach in your fruit smoothie.

- Rinse a can of chickpeas or cannellini beans and keep them in a covered bowl in the fridge for a quick spoonful or two of protein.

- Make at least one night a week meat-free, and experiment with bean-based dishes: burritos, rice and beans, Tuscan bean salad, tofu stir-fry, hummus, slow-cooked beans.

- Grill up vegetable kabobs next to your steak or fish.

- Store vegetables on the top shelf of your refrigerator instead of sticking them in the drawer so they'll be in your face, not tucked away.

At every meal, make your first question: How can I eat more vegetables at this meal? Yes, you can have a spinach, mushroom, tomato, broccoli omelette for breakfast—what a way to start your day! Soon it will become both habit and instinct—energizing, life-lengthening, time-creating choice!

Chapter Six

Take Care of Your Vehicle

Enjoying your life for a good long time has a lot to do with taking care of the actual nuts and bolts of your body—your bones and muscles—that get you from point A to point B with minimal pain and the maximum pleasure. And your skin, the largest organ of the body, is way more than simply tissue that holds it all together. The integumentary (skin) and musculoskeletal systems are the two aspects of health that most visibly reflect how we've taken care of ourselves over the years. When someone says, "She looks great!" or "She really let herself go," they're almost exclusively discussing the states of these two body systems.

Indeed, in countless ways, these systems (which, together, we'll call your vehicle) are not just about what we see on the outside. They are also a great reflection of the state of our interior physical health—and what our health future holds.

Fix It in 5
Prevent Age-Related Vehicle Damage

1. Wear sunscreen with an SPF of 30 on your face, ears, and exposed neck and shoulders every single day (and avoid burning on other areas of skin).
2. Drink six to eight glasses of water per day.
3. Floss!
4. Lift!
5. Jump!

Lately, our bodies' frames are not looking so good—we're seeing more and more fallout from our time-saving, body-wasting lifestyle, and it's now hitting us on a generational scale. A new study by the RAND Corporation found that the proportion of people ages 50 to 64 who needed help to do basic daily activities of living, such as getting in and out of bed, increased significantly between 1997 and 2007. While this group was hit hard by increases in disabilities due to depression, diabetes, and nervous system conditions, by far the most common reason for disability was musculoskeletal conditions. Many in this age group had problems walking for a quarter mile, standing up for 2 hours, and even just climbing a flight of stairs. While researchers could not pinpoint the reason for the increase, they said that many of the people over 50 who reported having disabilities had begun to experience health problems during their thirties and forties.

What types of problems? Arthritis, for one: Our risk of osteoarthritis increases by 9 to 13 percent for every 2 pounds gained above our ideal weight. Two pounds! Because the average person gains about a pound a year during midlife, you double your arthritis risk in the first 2 years, and the risk rises every year thereafter that you add more weight. Then consider all the other chronic, debilitating conditions that spring from too little exercise and too much cheap, easily accessible food, and it becomes a lot easier to see how we have fallen into a state of disrepair.

Discouraged? Don't be. Let's turn this trend around. Heck, you already have started on your way, simply by reading this book. We've discussed—and the RAND study demonstrates—that health issues can have a cumulative effect. But our bodies want to be healthy, and good health accumulates just as easily—maybe even more so, once we simply move in its direction. As we collect these 5-minute blocks of health, not only will they help us feel stronger and more energetic on the inside, they'll help us keep our vehicles on the road and moving fast.

A 5-Minute Tour of Your Bones, Muscles, and Skin

The frame of the body is the musculoskeletal system, an ingeniously constructed machine of bones, muscles, tendons, ligaments, joints, cartilage, and connective tissue. The bones are the base. They act as both the scaffolding for our bodies and as shields, protecting our fragile organs: The rib cage protects the lungs and the skull protects the brain.

But while bones are strong protectors, they are also malleable, at least at first. Babies' bones

```
I work at a computer all day, and sometimes
my wrists really hurt. How do I know if it's
just a sore wrist or carpal tunnel syndrome?
And if it is carpal tunnel, will I ever recover?
```

Dr. Drew says . . .

Carpal tunnel syndrome is one of those mysterious, scary diagnoses that people fear but don't really understand. They're most concerned that they might no longer be able to work if they develop the condition. But, thankfully, we have plenty of treatments for carpal tunnel.

Carpal tunnel syndrome occurs when the median nerve—the nerve that runs through the carpal tunnel of the wrist and connects with every finger except the little one—is pressed or squeezed at the wrist. It can be caused by illness, pregnancy, obesity, or injury from making repetitive motions. The nerve controls sensations to and from the palm side of the thumb and fingers, and symptoms include numbness, tingling, and burning in the palm and fingers. According to the NIH, women are three times more likely to suffer from it than men.

Doctors use specific tests to diagnose carpal tunnel syndrome, including Tinel's test, where the doctor taps on the median nerve to see if a shocklike sensation is felt. You can treat it by taking nonsteroidal anti-inflammatory drugs and wearing a wrist brace. In severe cases, a surgical treatment releases the pressure on the carpal ligament. Using a keyboard that has wrist supports and doing wrist and finger exercises can help prevent this syndrome. (The Arthritis Foundation recommends this exercise to help prevent carpal tunnel: Make a fist and then release hand and fan out fingers, stretching them as far as you can. Repeat five to 10 times.)

have growth plates that enable a tiny newborn to grow into an adult. And even as adults, our bones continue to change—they completely reform every 10 years, using calcium and vitamin D to strengthen themselves (which is why it's important to maintain adequate levels of these nutrients, even as we age).

Dem Bones, Dem Bones

For those who haven't attended medical school, mental images of bones were formed by the skeletons seen in Halloween decorations and the fossils of dinosaurs in museums. Consequently, many tend to think of bones as big, inanimate sticks held together by connective tissue at the joints—kind of like Tinkertoys of the body. But bones are incredibly alive: The outside layer of our bones is made up of proteins, like collagen, and the inner part stores the calcium and bone marrow, where blood cells are created. When we're kids, most of the bones in our bodies produce blood cells. Later, as adults, fewer and fewer of them do until just the large bones—the vertebrae (spinal column), sternum (breastbone), ribs, pelvis, and upper arm and leg bones—are still on the job. Yet when bones break, we don't feel pain in the bones themselves; instead, pain is transmitted by the nerves that surround them.

Joints connect bones to each other. Some move (like knees) and some don't (such as the joints between the plates of the skull). At a joint, the ends of the two bones that meet are covered in cartilage and surrounded by cells that produce fluid to reduce friction—your body's version of WD-40. This synovial fluid is filled with oxygen, nitrogen, and carbon dioxide, which form the gas bubbles that *pop!* loudly when you crack your knuckles. This pop is different from the one you hear when you crack your knee or ankle—those are caused by the tendon snapping back into its original position. And the cracking sound you don't want to hear is closer to a grinding sound, which is a result of arthritis; it means you've lost smooth cartilage in the joint, and what you're hearing is bone-on-bone friction. You might hear it—although you don't want to!—in any of the three basic types of moving joints: hinges (the knees and elbows), pivot joints (which move the head from side to side), and ball and socket joints (the hips and shoulders).

Intermingled with all these bones and joints are the muscles—more than 650 of them, which together can make up half of our body weight. Connecting the muscles to the bones are tendons, which act like puppet strings, enabling the muscles to move the bones. We have several types of muscle tissue.

The skeletal muscles are responsible for our everyday body movements and hold the skeleton together. These muscles are capable of either flexing or extending, and the body cleverly places one of each type in pairs. For example, when you curl a dumbbell, the extender muscle straightens out the arm and the flexor brings it back in.

The smooth muscles, which we don't even realize are working, are controlled automatically by the brain to perform basic body functions such as digestion, breathing, and blood flow.

(We have another type of muscle that's not part of our musculoskeletal vehicle, but, rather, composes its engine: the cardiac muscles that form the heart have the same consistency as skeletal muscles but move involuntarily like smooth muscles.)

(Don't) Give Them a Break

Injury is probably the greatest enemy of the musculoskeletal system, especially as our bodies spend a longer time kicking around on the planet. Protecting our bones and muscles from injury will be key later on to a longer life. Increasing muscle strength and preserving bone mass, which many of our 5-minute fixes are designed to do, will help us do just that. Most of these same fixes can also help us stave off some of the diseases that can attack the musculoskeletal system, such as arthritis.

Arthritis is inflammation in the joints that causes stiffness or pain that can be mild, but can also be very serious and debilitating. Now, the incidence of arthritis does increase with age, but there definitely are some things we can do to help prevent it. Being overweight increases the risk and also the severity of arthritis, so managing your weight will lower your arthritis risk, too. You get one type of arthritis—gout—primarily from eating and drinking foods high in the chemical compound purine (such as most meats, some seafood, and too much beer!), not drinking enough water, and packing on the pounds—all of which may exacerbate a genetic predisposition or an enzyme deficiency that makes it hard for your body to break down purines. Gout is like having kidney stones, but in a joint. Urate crystals, which form because there is too much uric acid in the body, collect in the joint (most commonly the one at the base of the big toe), and it can be extremely painful. Thankfully (because we all are busy people!), several 5-minute health fixes we can do to avoid gout—drink less alcohol, eat more veggies and less meat, get more exercise, and drink more water—definitely fall into the category of health multitaskers that are good for several things that might ail us. Yes, they are definitely time-creators.

Keep It Together

Although it is not part of the musculoskeletal system, the skin is the largest organ in the body, surrounding the muscles and protecting everything inside the body, keeping everything in place and acting as a barrier. Our skin has three layers, the outer layer (epidermis), the middle layer (dermis), and the bottom layer (sometimes called the hypodermis, it is composed of fat), and each has its own special purpose. In one way, humans are like snakes: Our skin is constantly regenerating. New cells form in the bottom layer and make their way to the top as the old ones eventually flake off. (Perhaps some of us are like snakes in more than one way, but that's a discussion for another day.)

Within the epidermis are melanin cells, which give the skin its color and is also where our sweat lives. That surface—the epidermis—is where the action happens.

The dermis—the skin's middle layer—sends messages to the brain when you touch something—anything—and the brain interprets that sensation. It could be something wildly unpleasant (recall from Chapter 3 the hot stove that makes our nerves scream, "Hot!") that puts our muscles into action. But it could also be something way more pleasurable, like feeling a warm breeze on a spring day or stroking the soft cheek of a baby—or, some other, skin-on-skin sensations, but we'll let you use your imagination on that one.

With the help of the sweat glands, the skin works as a thermostat to gauge the outside temperature and help keep the body at a steady 98.6°F or so. If it's hot outside, the body brings warm blood to the surface of your skin, you get flushed, and your sweat glands release moisture, cooling off the surface of your skin as it evaporates. If you are cold, blood vessels in the dermis narrow to bring the warm blood inward and muscles at the base of your hair follicles contract—and you get goose bumps.

As much as we crave tons of time in that bright, warm weather, one of the major enemies of the skin is the sun. While 30 minutes a day in the bright sunshine can help us generate vital vitamin D, when those intense ultraviolet rays that beat down from the sun land directly on our skin and our cells interact with that radiation, they can start to grow irregularly, resulting in skin cancer.

Now, there are many different types of cancer, some of which are more dangerous than others. When epidermal cells start to grow irregularly, they can develop into basal or squamous cell cancers, which can be very treatable. However, when the skin pigment cells, called melanocytes, begin to proliferate in the deeper layers of the epidermis, they can morph into the dreaded melanoma—a potentially deadly form of cancer that can spread throughout the body,

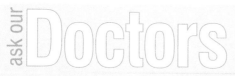

I've been thinking about plastic surgery
for years. How do I know if I'm really ready?
And what can I do to prepare myself?

Dr. Drew says . . .

To be honest, I wish more patients would be this thoughtful about plastic surgery. Though my fellow surgeons and I are skilled physicians, we can't help you heal if you are doing this for the wrong reasons. To prevent any regrets or ill-advised surgeries, please be sure to follow these dos and don'ts before you commit to any procedure.

DOS

1. **DO do your research on the doctor.** As I've said on the show before, some people spend more time researching the purchase of a flat-screen TV than they do checking out their own doctors. Don't be afraid to press for details from your doctor:

   - Does he do a lot of these procedures?
   - Is she a board-certified plastic surgeon?
   - Can you see photos of his results?
   - Can you meet with any of her patients?
   - Is the facility accredited?

A no to any of these questions should automatically disqualify that doctor from your consideration.

and a major reason why dermatologists insist that we wear sunscreen. Of course, the sun can also dry out your skin, and a lifetime spent sitting in the sun can result in dry, thin, less elastic skin that becomes creased with wrinkles. We love your baby face, which is why we want you to invest in a good hat, slather on SPF 30 or higher sunscreen, and avoid cigarettes—nothing ages a person's face faster than smoking or tanning.

Don't get us wrong—we don't want you to barricade yourselves indoors and never see the

2. **DO have realistic goals.** Realize that this is real surgery: You will be given general anesthesia and a person with a knife will cut into your body. No surgery is without risks; carefully consider the potential complications.

DON'TS

1. **DON'T rush into it.** Make sure the procedure is right for you. Be clear about what your surgical goals are. What do you want to change? How likely is it that the result will be close to your ideal? Ask all of your questions before surgery, so you're fully prepared and you know exactly what you are getting yourself into.

2. **DON'T have surgery for the wrong reasons.** Plastic surgery is not something you do for your boyfriend, your husband, or your job—you should do it only for yourself. Don't expect surgery to change your entire life. Understand that changing something on the outside is not necessarily going to make you happier on the inside.

3. **DON'T request unnatural results or procedures.** Be realistic about the body type you were born with; if you are a petite, 5-foot-tall woman, be wary of a doctor who believes you should get size D implants. Sadly, some doctors are willing to perform procedures that aren't right for your body simply to make money, or to give you a look that they think is right.

4. **DON'T let cost be the determining factor of which surgeon you select.** If I had my way, there'd be a "Buyer, beware" sign in every plastic surgeon's office as a visual reminder that you usually get what you pay for in aesthetic surgery. You will have to live with your face and body and the results of this surgery for the rest of your life. Invest wisely.

sun again. We humans need the sun to thrive, just like we need fresh air and water. If we only become smarter about our sun exposure—using a combination of 5-minute fixes and a good dose of common sense—we can delight in the warmth, soak in enough healthy rays, and still avoid the degree of exposure that's linked with wrinkles and one of the deadliest forms of cancer. Combine these changes with others that protect your bones and muscles, and your vehicle will be the nicest one on the road for years to come.

5-Minute Fixes
for a Lifetime of Bone, Muscle, and Skin Health

Move it or lose it: They're words to live by. And as we've seen, this rule is one of the best time-creators around. If you're reading this book, chances are that your peak muscle- and bone-building years are done and your body is straddling the divide between youthful, take-it-for-granted health and beauty and getting-up-there, wish-I-knew-what-I-had-when-I-had-it regrets about not having taken care of yourself properly. Well, dear reader, hear this: It is never too late. People in their nineties can increase their muscle mass with three-times-a-week weight training. If you're only half that age (or less) you need to seize the day and get to work, now! While you're at it, try a few more of these 5-minute fixes, which are all about maintaining your ride and keeping it at its shiny, happy, healthy best.

Suck on an antiaging frozen pop. Liz Vaccariello, former editor-in-chief of *Prevention* magazine, suggested this tasty treat to help you look younger and achieve better health. The antiaging popsicle contains carrot juice, pomegranate juice, and 100 percent cherry juice that is free of red dye and corn syrup. Each juice provides benefits that help you look younger and achieve better health.

> **Cherry juice:** In addition to containing high levels of antioxidants, cherries have anti-inflammatory and antiaging properties, and they have been shown to help fight cancer and heart disease.

> **Pomegranate juice:** Like cherry juice, pomegranate juice is also high in antioxidants. Research shows that it can lower cholesterol and reduce blood pressure, as well.

> **Carrot juice:** The beta-carotene and vitamin A in carrot juice can help reduce wrinkles and dry skin and fight free radicals. Research shows that carrots may also reduce the risk of age-related macular degeneration, a leading cause of blindness.

I'm almost 50 and have never taken a calcium supplement. Are my bones doomed to crumble into dust? What can I do now to make them as strong as possible?

Dr. Lisa says . . .

It's never too late to take steps to guard against brittle bones and fractures. These steps will help:

Make a commitment to calcium. You need 1,200 milligrams per day starting at age 50. How you get it is up to you. Three servings of low-fat or fat-free dairy products will get you close. Adding other calcium-containing foods such as spinach, kale, whole wheat bread, canned salmon with the bones, even almonds can help. You could also take calcium supplements to hit your daily target. Take up to 600 milligrams of calcium at a time; your body can't absorb more than that from a dose. Best bet: A calcium supplement that also contains vitamin D for better absorption.

Get your D and K. Both help with calcium absorption and maintaining bone health. Aim for 400 to 600 IU (international units) of vitamin D a day—from a separate supplement, in your calcium tablet, or even from 15 to 30 minutes of exposure to sunshine twice a week if you live in the southern half of the United States. Many experts think the recommended dose of vitamin D is too low (visit www.vitamindcouncil.org for more information). Do your research and decide how much is right for you—but get some! You'll also need 90 to 120 micrograms a day of vitamin K—the amount in a serving or two of kale, broccoli, spinach, Brussels sprouts, or dark green lettuce such as romaine.

Move! Weight-bearing exercises like brisk walking, dancing, strength training, walking up and down stairs, jogging, and tennis put stress on bones that helps make them stronger and denser. Strong muscles also increase your balance and flexibility, so you're less likely to have a bone-fracturing fall.

Ask your doctor about a bone density scan. A scan is recommended for all women when they reach 50 (or when menopause starts), but you may want to have one sooner if you have any risk factors for brittle bones. These include having a family or personal history of bone fracture due to brittle bones, smoking, regularly having more than one alcoholic drink a day, or taking oral corticosteroid drugs (such as those for asthma), as well as having rheumatoid arthritis.

WHAT YOUR BODY'S TRYING TO TELL YOU: NAILS, SKIN, AND HAIR

Dull hair, brittle nails, sallow skin. Do you just need a new brand of shampoo or soap, or is it a medical condition that merits a trip to the doctor's office? Here's what your body is trying to tell you.

Symptoms: Lengthwise (vertical) or crosswise (horizontal) ridges in your nails

What it could mean: Sometimes just aging, but noticeable vertical ridges—running from the base to the tip of your nail—could be a sign of rheumatoid arthritis, peripheral vascular disease, or—if there's a large ridge running down the middle of your nail, a protein, folic acid, or iron deficiency. Horizontal ridges that run from side to side are usually a sign they were formed during a serious illness in your past, possibly a severe infection, heart attack, major surgery, or cancer treatment.

What to do: See your doctor for evaluation of any troubling ridges.

Symptoms: Tiny, vertical white lines in your nails

What it could mean: Diabetes, a thyroid disorder, a vitamin B deficiency

What to do: Ask your doctor to take a look at your next appointment; in the meantime, be sure you're taking good care of your health—get regular exercise; eat a healthy diet full of produce, whole grains, and lean protein (skip sweets, packaged snacks, and high-fat foods); and take a multivitamin.

Symptoms: Thin, brittle nails

What it could mean: Your nails may be too dry (thanks to low humidity and the drying effects of indoor heat). If your nails feel soft and are so thin they're breaking, it may be the opposite problem: They may be getting wet too often due to dishwashing, cleaning, or exposure to chemicals or even nail polish remover. Rarely, thin, brittle nails are a sign of thinning bones (osteopenia) or a thyroid disorder.

What to do: Moisturize with a lotion that contains lanolin or an alpha hydroxy acid. Wear rubber gloves when cleaning or washing dishes. Switch to an acetone-free nail polish remover. If your toenails and fingernails stay thin and brittle, mention it to your doctor at your next appointment.

Symptoms: Nails that curve dramatically toward or away from your skin

What it could mean: An upward curve could be a sign of diabetes or an iron deficiency. A severe downward curve could be a sign of a kidney or thyroid disorder or psoriasis.

What to do: Call your doctor for an evaluation.

Symptoms: Tired-looking skin

What it could mean: Dehydration

What to do: Be sure to drink six to eight 8-ounce glasses of water per day, and even a little more if you're exercising or the weather is hot.

Symptoms: A dull complexion that lacks a healthy glow

What it could mean: Lack of exercise

What to do: Aim for a half hour of activity on most days of the week. It's okay to split it up into two or three shorter sessions (like a couple of 10-minute walks), too. Exercise increases blood circulation, making your skin look healthier and younger.

Symptoms: Sallow, yellowish skin

What it could mean: Jaundice—possibly due to a liver problem, bile duct blockage, or a mild genetic condition called Gilbert's syndrome. In jaundice, the skin and whites of the eyes turn yellow. Yellowish-orange skin may simply be a sign that you've eaten a lot of foods containing beta-carotene, such as carrots and cantaloupe. In that case, the whites of the eyes will remain white.

What to do: Choose a wider variety of fruits and vegetables if you think you've been eating too much yellow and orange produce. If the whites of your eyes also look yellowish, call your doctor for an evaluation.

Symptoms: Thinning or lifeless hair, or losing more hair in your brush or comb, on your pillow in the morning, or in the shower after shampooing

What it could mean: Most—about 90 percent—of hair loss is simply due to genetics. Stress, some anticlotting medications and blood pressure drugs, and a low iron blood level can also be the cause. If your eyebrows are also thinning—especially if you're losing hair on the outer third of your eyebrows—it could mean you have an underactive thyroid (hypothyroidism, covered in greater detail in Chapter 7).

What to do: Mention it to your doctor at your next visit. Call for an appointment if hair loss begins suddenly, becomes dramatically worse, or if you lose hair in patches.

Pour equal portions of each juice into a pitcher or blender and stir briefly. Pour into popsicle molds (available at discount stores for less than $10). Or, to enjoy several small doses during the day, use an ice cube tray: Pour in the juice, spread plastic wrap over the top, secure the plastic with a large rubber band, and then poke toothpicks through the plastic into the juice and freeze. In a few hours, you'll have mini-popsicle sticks. **Time spent:** 5 minutes to blend and store in the freezer; 5 minutes to savor and enjoy

Swipe on sunscreen before you swipe on deodorant. Doing so will not only help you remember to use sunscreen on a daily basis, it will also give the sunscreen time to set and dry before you either apply your makeup or hit the great outdoors. Many people wait until they're out in the sun before applying sunscreen—and then they blame any resulting itchy or blotchy reactions on the fact that their skin "hates sunscreen." If your skin is already hot and sweaty, your pores are more open than normal and more sunscreen will be absorbed than may be advisable. It's possible that your skin may be sensitive to just one of the typically many ingredients in your sunscreen, rather than to sunscreens in general.

Check out the Environmental Working Group's database of personal care products, Skin Deep (www.cosmeticsdatabase.com). You'll find almost 1,800 products that have an SPF rating, all searchable according to their ingredients—such as para-aminobenzoic acid (PABA) or oxybenzone—and their potential toxicity. If you are allergic to a particular compound, you can search for recommended products without that particular offender. Also, some prescriptions, such as antibiotics and acne medications, can make your skin more sensitive to sun damage. Next time you fill your prescription, ask your doctor or pharmacist to recommend a brand of sunscreen that will not interact with your current drug regimen. But most important of all: Just put it on! **Time spent:** 4 minutes researching the best sunscreen option online; 1 minute applying sunscreen every morning

Or steal some of your baby's butt cream. Over-the-counter diaper rash cream that contains zinc oxide and aloe vera moisturizes and repairs your face, and it is ideal for dry,

My mom always told me to put butter on a burn,
but that just seems gross. What's the real story?

Dr. Drew says . . .

You're right. Besides being disgusting, butter on a burn not only traps the heat, causing further discomfort, but also could easily cause infection.

Another mistake people make is that they immediately submerge the burned skin in ice—bad idea. Ice is as caustic as heat and can cause frostbite, which is actually similar to a burn. Instead, try these steps:

1. Submerge the burn in cool water (or let cool water run over it) for 10 to 15 minutes, then gently treat it with a cool compress.

2. Apply aloe vera (for superficial burns, such as sunburn) or a triple antibiotic cream.

3. If you have a blister, don't pop it! If the burn is severe, your doctor may pop the blister under sterile conditions, but under no circumstances should this be done at home.

4. Cover the wound with a nonstick bandage. (Normal gauze can stick to the wound and, when you try to remove it later, it will rip the top layer of the burn right off. Ouch.)

5. If you have some pain or swelling, take ibuprofen to help relieve some of the inflammation.

flaky skin. Used in many skin preparations, zinc oxide has a mild astringent and soothing effect. These types of creams can be used to treat painful, itchy, or moist skin conditions. And, bonus, with zinc oxide's ultraviolet-blocking power, they double as sunblocks! Products that include aloe vera benefit from its nutrients, vitamins, active compounds, essential minerals, and amino acids that reduce inflammation. **Time spent:** 1 minute every morning putting it on

Warm up to warm up. One of the biggest mistakes novice exercisers make is stretching cold muscles. Michele Olson, PhD, FACSM, professor of exercise science at the Human Performance Laboratory at Auburn University in Montgomery, Alabama, recommends this warmup: When you head out for a walk, to increase the blood flow to your legs and get your heart rate up, begin walking slowly, taking long steps. Then take shorter steps at a faster speed, and then alternate these two patterns five to seven times for 2 minutes each. Also, alternate swinging and crossing your arms in front of your chest with making arm circles while you do this walking exercise. Your arms and chest are very important in all types of exercise, so they need the increased blood flow, too. When you start to feel a few beads of sweat breaking, that's your cue to speed up and do your regular workout. Save the stretching until after exercise, when your muscles and joints are well lubricated and more pliable, so you can stretch more comfortably and with less risk of injury. **Time spent:** approximately 5 minutes to warm up before your regular walk or run

After drinking coffee, dry brush your teeth—but wait 20 minutes. After drinking coffee, tea, or any other acidic beverage, rinse your mouth with water and then wait 20 minutes before you put a brush anywhere near your teeth. Otherwise, you could be brushing the enamel off your teeth while it's still soft from the acid—and once the enamel is gone, it's gone for good. Dry brushing after 20 minutes will reduce tartar buildup by 60 percent and the risk of bleeding gums by half. Then follow up with "wet" brushing—with traditional toothpaste—for that minty clean feeling. Invest in soft-bristle toothbrushes for everyone in your household for every sink in the house—the kitchen, the half bath next to the TV room, and, of course, your own bathroom. You'll never be more than a few steps away from a clean mouth after a meal. **Time spent:** 1 minute for dry brushing; 1 minute for "wet" brushing (with toothpaste)

And be wary of tartar control toothpaste. To go with your toothbrush in every bathroom, stock up on minitubes of toothpaste as well, but you may want to steer clear of tartar control formulas. If you are a vigorous brusher, their added abrasive agents can contribute to receding gums, leaving your mouth (and, therefore, your whole body!) more vulnerable to germs. Even more troubling is the use of the antibacterial triclosan in toothpaste. While it's been proven to help reduce gingivitis, recent research suggests that, when combined with the chlorine in standard municipal tap water, triclosan can react to form the potentially cancer-causing gas chloroform. Also, triclosan's chemical structure is similar to that of both the banned anti-miscarriage drug diethylstilbestrol (often called DES) and the controversial plastic additive bisphenol A, which act like hormones in the body. Play it old school: Get plain fluoride paste, without all the fancy bells and whistles. **Time spent:** 5 minutes to read labels in the toothpaste aisle

Get on the Mole Patrol. The most important gift you can give your skin is your attention. We'd like nothing better than for you to get to know your skin so well that you'll instantly recognize anything that's troubling. The American Academy of Dermatology recommends that you do a thorough self-exam to get to know your skin's quirks.

- Using a mirror, inspect the front and back of your body, then lift your arms and inspect your sides.
- Bend your elbows and examine the entire lengths of your arms, hands, and palms.
- Inspect the fronts and backs of your legs, the tops and bottoms of your feet, and between your toes.
- Grab a hand mirror to look at the back of your neck and your scalp. Move your hair out of the way to inspect the scalp.
- Use the hand mirror to also check your back and buttocks.

If you have a significant number of moles, you might consider enlisting your spouse or a close friend to photograph your body in exactly this systematic way. You can keep these photos digitally on your computer for reference, in case you notice any changes. The appearance of new moles is not that worrisome (although you should try to prevent them by using sunscreen

BEAUTY RX: AT-HOME BEAUTY

Every day, we're becoming more and more aware of the dangers of some of the chemicals used in our personal care products. From the innocuous-sounding "fragrance" to the endocrine-disrupting phthalates, our still-limited awareness of what we're putting on our skin could be putting us in danger. What's the solution? Create your own beauty products—usually for a fraction of the cost of high-end beauty items. Kym Douglas, TV personality and best-selling coauthor with syndicated entertainment writer Cindy Pearlman of *The Beauty Cookbook: Over 200 Recipes to Make Your Kitchen Your Own Personal Spa—for Your Face, Your Body, and Your Hair*, came on the show to share some of her homemade Hollywood beauty secrets. Try these yourself—some are good enough to eat!

DRY SKIN SMOOTHIE

INGREDIENTS

- 1 **banana**
- 1 **cup plain yogurt**
- 1 **tablespoon honey**
- 2 **tablespoons rolled oats**

WHAT TO DO

In a blender, puree the banana and then add the yogurt, honey, and oats and mix well. Smooth the mixture over your damp face (and, if there's any extra, put some on your hair and rinse as instructed on the opposite page). Let it soak in for 15 minutes and then rinse with warm water. Your face will feel hydrated in no time!

INGREDIENT BENEFITS

BANANA

- Contains tryptophan, a rich amino acid that is known to be extremely beneficial for hair and skin
- Contains potassium and vitamins A, B, C, and E, which soften the hair shaft and skin
- Contains rich natural oils and carbohydrates, which are beneficial for the skin

YOGURT

- Works as a natural moisturizer
- Has high zinc content that helps to clear blemishes
- Contains lactic acid, a natural skin smoother that also reduces pore size, improves overall skin texture, and gives you a healthy glow

HONEY

- Has antibacterial properties that help calm acne and breakouts
- Brightens and energizes the skin (the darker the honey, the purer it is)
- Is a natural moisturizer that was used by the Egyptians and Romans

ROLLED OATS

- Gently scrub sensitive skin
- Have healing properties

BAGEL HEAD CONDITIONER

INGREDIENTS

1 **egg**

2 **tablespoons cream cheese**

2 **tablespoons butter**

2 **tablespoons water**

WHAT TO DO

Mix the egg, cream cheese, butter, and water in a food processor or with a whisk. Slather the mixture on your hair and work it through with a wide-toothed comb. Use extra on the ends. Leave it on for 15 minutes, then rinse it out with warm water. Do this once a week to get silky, healthy-looking hair. It's ideal for repairing damaged processed hair!

Continued

INGREDIENT BENEFITS

EGG

- Rich in vitamins A, D, and E as well as several B vitamins, all of which are good for hair
- Increases sebum production, which oils dry hair and prevents dandruff, with vitamin A
- Helps hair grow with vitamin D
- Increases the scalp's oxygen-absorption capacity with vitamin E
- Increases hemoglobin's oxygen-carrying capacity and improves blood circulation with B vitamins
- Contains fatty acids that make hair shiny and manageable, improve skin structure, and lessen dandruff, hair loss, psoriasis, and flaky scalp

CREAM CHEESE AND BUTTER

- Stimulate the roots of the hair and the hair follicles and promote growth with whey, or milk plasma

or thoroughly covering yourself when you're in the sun). But keep a particularly close eye on existing moles to watch for any changes in the ABCDEs:

- Asymmetry? If it's uneven or lopsided, that's a sign you have to go see your doctor.
- Border irregularity? Watch to make sure they're not scalloped or notched.
- Color? Are there any variations in color within the mole? Does it contain more than one shade of tan, brown, red, or black? Does it bleed easily?
- Diameter? The entire mole should be smaller than six millimeters, the diameter of a pencil eraser.
- Evolving? Have you noticed any change?

If you notice any changes, share your images and observations with your dermatologist. Work this mole patrol into your weekly grooming routine, perhaps doing it between giving

PINEAPPLE PEDICURE

INGREDIENT

1 one-inch slice fresh pineapple

WHAT TO DO

Remove any old polish with nail polish remover. Wash and dry your hands thoroughly. Rub the pineapple slice over your nails and cuticles. When you're done coating each nail, allow the juice to work its way into the nail beds for 1 to 2 minutes. Wipe away the excess juice, but don't wash or rinse off your toes. Using a damp washcloth, gently push back the cuticles. Do this once a week to clean and brighten your toenails and remove dead cuticle particles.

INGREDIENT BENEFITS

PINEAPPLE

- Contains bromelain, a protein-digesting enzyme
- Has anti-inflammatory properties
- Contains chemicals that interfere with the growth of tumor cells

yourself a pedicure and plucking your eyebrows. **Time spent:** 15 minutes for first photography session, then 5 minutes once a week to give yourself a thorough once-over

Cut a lemon in half. And rub a half on each elbow. As both men and women get older, the skin on our elbows and knees can get a bit darker. The vitamin C in lemons is a natural skin lightener. If the skin is also a bit rough and scaly, put the pulp and juice from each half of the lemon in a bowl and mix it with coffee grounds (whatever is left over from one pot of coffee), a natural exfoliant. Using both together at the same time will let you scrub away old dead skin while you brighten the newly revealed, fresh skin below. **Time spent:** 2 minutes on each elbow

Treat your stinky feet to some tea. Are your dogs not only barking, but stinking up the joint? Most chronic foot odor is caused by bacteria. To give your feet a treat you'll enjoy as well, brew up a big pot of black tea and pour it into a foot bath. Let the tea cool until you're able to comfortably submerge your feet in it. Sit back, relax, and soak your feet for 30 minutes. Repeat the process every day for a week. The tannic acid in the tea will kill the bacteria and also close the sweat pores in your feet. **Time spent:** 5 minutes to brew the tea; 30 minutes a day to relax and enjoy

Drink an extra glass of milk with your salty food. Calcium is very important to your bones, but certain foods can upset the balance of calcium in the body, such as those containing too much caffeine or protein. But salt is particularly troublesome, not only because we Americans tend to eat so much of it, but also because it is very efficient at speeding up this calcium depletion. Studies on women suggest that every additional 1,000 mg of salt per day a woman eats increases her bone loss by 1 percent per year—unless she can compensate by adding more calcium to her diet. Why take chances? Shoot for calcium extra credit—get four servings of low-fat dairy per day, especially if you're a salt fiend. **Time spent:** 3 minutes to drink an extra glass of fat-free or 1% milk

Step away from the mirror. For some of us, squeezing zits is a habit that's as hard to break as biting your nails or smoking. But try to resist the temptation. If you can't, and you have bacteria on your fingers when you dig in, you'll cause scabs and scars on your face. Think about it this way: Acne is basically an abscess—you're performing surgery on your face with your dirty fingers.

A zit starts below the skin when sebum, a fluid naturally produced by sebaceous glands, can't get to the surface because a pore is blocked. Zits come in two forms—blackheads and whiteheads. A blackhead, or black comedo, is open to the air, whereas a whitehead, or white comedo, is closed. A dermatologist will use a comedo extractor to release the pus, the white blood cells, and dead tissue inside the abscess.

But you're not a dermatologist. Instead of picking, treat both types of zits with acne medications like salicylic acid, retinoic acid, and benzoyl peroxide. If you've tried to keep your hands off but can't help yourself, try this popping alternative: Put a warm compress on your zit for a few minutes, followed by a cold wet chamomile tea bag, also for a few minutes. This will

I hear about different degrees of burns,
but I really have no idea what that means.
Is first degree the worst, or is it third?

Dr. Drew says . . .

You'd be surprised how many people have this exact question for me all the time.

First-Degree Burn: This type occurs when only the outer later of skin is burned. It is the least serious type of burn and can cause the skin to turn red, with slight swelling and some pain. A sunburn is a first-degree burn.

Second-Degree Burn: This type of burn injures the outer layer of skin and extends into the second layer, which is called the dermis. It can cause the skin to turn red and blisters to develop and result in severe pain and swelling.

Third-Degree Burn: This is the most serious type of burn, and it affects all three layers of the skin. It can char the skin or cause a dry, whitish appearance and can result in permanent tissue damage. If a person is extremely badly burned, he or she may require a skin graft.

soothe the pimple, open it up, and even kill some of the bacteria inside the pore, decreasing inflammation. But seriously, try to restrain yourself—for your skin's sake. **Time spent:** hopefully you'll save time by not popping your zits, but if you do give in to temptation, 5 minutes to use the chamomile option

Find out about fillers. If you've been curious about facial fillers and want to know what's what, why wait? Temporary fillers—such as hyaluronic acid and collagen—give you the opportunity to fill in everything from lines to scars to severe folds in your facial skin. The filler material is absorbed by your body in 6 to 8 months. Or, you might choose to use your

Medicine, 16 Uses

Botox

If you've ever watched the show, you know that we—especially Dr. Drew—are big fans of Botox. This modern marvel of medicine started out as a toxic by-product—botulinum toxin—of a type of bacterium, *Clostridium botulinum*. But since it was introduced for medical use more than 20 years ago, doctors in many medical fields have found a truly amazing variety of uses for it.

The most popular use, of course, is the one that relieves wrinkles. When doctors give us tiny injections of this nerve poison, they're actually giving our faces a little vacation. Muscles that are usually used to frown or scowl don't move, so they don't get a chance to form wrinkles or lines. A recent study from the University of Wisconsin–Madison found Botox may actually go a step further—in addition to hiding those negative emotions, it may even help prevent you from feeling them! In 40 people who'd received Botox injections in their corrugator muscle, the muscle between your eyebrows that crinkles up when you frown, researchers found a small but distinct change in their ability to recognize angry or sad statements as such. After the injections, the subjects had no trouble identifying happy statements, but they were briefly befuddled by angry or sad sentences.

The researchers suggest this effect was

own fat, harvested from your belly, thighs, or buttocks, to fill out hollow cheeks, facial lines, or even your lips. (Many patients prefer this as a more natural option.) Of course, the least invasive and most temporary option is Botox injections. This option doesn't actually fill the lines, but rather paralyzes certain muscles in your face so they can take a breather and relax a bit, allowing the skin to flatten out and not be cramped into a wrinkle all day. Its results last about 3 months.

Depending on your budget, your goals, and your lifestyle, there are many options. Go to the Consumer Guide to Plastic Surgery (http://www.yourplasticsurgeryguide.com/surgeons) to search for the name of a board-certified plastic surgeon in your area. **Time spent:** 2 minutes to locate a local doctor and 3 minutes to set up an appointment

proof of the "facial feedback hypothesis," which holds that once you feel an emotion and register it on your face, the signals from your facial expression shoot back to the brain to reinforce the emotion. This area of research is still developing—as are many other areas of Botox usage. Recently, the FDA required Botox to add a "black box" warning for a rare but potentially serious complication, migration of the toxin beyond the injection site—but many doctors agree that the quantities used for cosmetic purposes have nearly zero risks.

Here are just a few uses for Botox that have been *suggested* (not necessarily FDA approved) in the past few years.

1. Reduce facial wrinkles in forehead, around the eyes, and between the eyebrows (these are frown lines, of course!)
2. Relieve small bunions and their associated pain
3. Relieve uncontrolled blinking
4. Correct lazy or crossed eyes
5. Relieve head tilting, neck pain, and neck muscle spasms (cervical dystonia)
6. Ease migraines
7. Calm an overactive bladder
8. Reduce surgical pain and other types of pain
9. Prevent ringing in the ears
10. Control drooling and other symptoms of cerebral palsy
11. Stop chronic pelvic pain
12. Relieve digestive problems related to diabetes
13. Control spasms related to multiple sclerosis, trauma, or stroke
14. Relieve jaw tension
15. Reduce excessive sweating
16. Possibly reduce angry or sad emotions

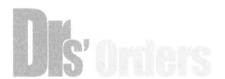

Drs' Orders

for Bone and Muscle Health: Jump! (And do other high-impact, weight-bearing exercises, too)

It's official—we don't exercise nearly enough. But we can change, and it will not take a million years to get the job done. It will take just 5 minutes at a time, here and there, to make a tremendous difference.

As a society, we need to make big changes, and the new approach needs to begin in childhood. According to the CDC, only half of those ages 12 to 21 exercise vigorously on a regular basis, and 14 percent don't exercise at all. We've lost the playing, recess games, and endless bike rides through the neighborhood that used to tire us out as kids and make us sleep like rocks. And our kids are paying a steep price. And by the time those less-active kids become adults, the consequences of this country's health condition are really going to hit the fan.

For their sake and ours, we need to jump to it. Exercise-intervention studies in girls suggest that relatively short periods of the right kinds of exercise can stimulate hip and spine bone growth. The most powerful type of exercise? Jumping, especially when done on a hard surface. You can guess what we say to that: Break out the jump rope! Try a few moves and ask your kid to show you a few more. Let him or her jump off the swing or swing down out of the tree before landing with a thud. Every time they jump from moderate heights (about 20 inches), they're building bone in the most efficient way possible.

(One caveat: Repetitive impact—such as regularly jogging or running on hard surfaces— can lead to shin splints, a painful but temporary overstrain injury.)

But do you think these results are only for kids? They're not. It turns out that our skeletons really love strength training and short bouts of high-load impact activity such as skipping and jumping, both of which improve muscle strength as well as bone mass. The more weight-bearing, intense activity we do, the more we can protect our bodies against the natural ravages of time. But while sarcopenia, the involuntary loss of skeletal muscle mass and function, was once thought to be induced solely by age, we now know that we can do a lot to combat it. As we get older, the enzymes in our muscle cells' mitochondria naturally start to slow down, but exercise can increase their activity. In addition, blood levels of our muscle-building hormones, human growth hormone and testosterone, wane as we get older, but exercise can help keep their levels higher.

And while we no longer really build bone as adults, exercise can certainly help us protect and defend what we have. Muscle-building exercise has been shown to improve the strength and physical performance of even frail nursing home residents, reducing their risk of broken

DOCTOR, DOCTOR, GIMME THE NEWS:
FLAT IS FANTASTIC FOR FEET

After decades of advice that urged us to protect our knees by wearing "supportive" shoes—are they always ugly?—with plenty of arch arc, new research from Rush University Medical Center has found that slackers' favorites shoes might work just as well. It turns out that sneakers with flexible soles and even flip-flops might be easier on the knees than clogs or special walking shoes.

In a study published in the journal *Arthritis Care and Research*, author Najia Shakoor, MD, a rheumatologist at Rush, and her colleagues analyzed the gaits of 31 patients with symptoms of osteoarthritis in the Rush Motion Analysis Laboratory. The researchers studied them while they walked barefoot and in four popular shoe types: clogs (the type often worn by doctors and nurses), stability-control athletic shoes, flat sneakers with flexible soles, and flip-flops. Surprisingly, Dr. Shakoor found that the clogs and stability shoes caused a 15 percent higher load on the knee than walking in flat shoes, flip-flops, or barefoot. This finding followed Dr. Shakoor and her team's earlier research that found barefoot walking was better for the body because the natural flex of the foot softens the impact on the knees. Placing a high stress load on the knee is a key factor affecting both the severity and the progression of osteoarthritis, the most common form of arthritis and a significant source of impairment in the quality of life as we get older, so anything we can do to relieve that load is a good thing.

If you are drawn to high heel shoes, you're in worse luck than supportive-shoe wearers. Shoes with heels higher than 3 inches place many times more pressure on your feet and disrupt your center of gravity. If you like to wear heels, try to keep them to 2 inches or lower, and be sure to stretch your calves during the day. And as soon as you get home, ditch them for your slippers or flip-flops, or just go naked. Your feet, that is.

bones by improving balance, mobility, and speed, all of which prevent falls—or at least make their effects much, much less dangerous. Several large studies have reported that exercise leads to 10 percent fewer falls, while balance training leads to 17 percent fewer falls. Men in their eighties and nineties who start to exercise can see their strength increase by more than 100 percent—you can't get much better than that!

Okay, it's settled. Exercise it is. But how do you incorporate it into your daily life? What if you can't afford a gym membership? Bring the gym to your place! We asked Crunch Gym personal fitness trainer Alycia Perrin to devise a home workout that will fit anyone's budget. She recommends that you first gather some very basic equipment.

- Stability ball: $20
- Two dumbbells (5 pounders for beginners, 8 pounders for intermediates): $15
- Medium resistance level resistance band: $10
- Jump rope: $5

TOTAL = $50

Alycia's Home Workout Tips

JUMP ROPE

Do some simple rope skipping to raise your heart rate, burn calories, and warm up muscles—and help protect those bones. A 15-minute session can burn more than 150 calories!

STABILITY BALL

Do crunches on a stability ball. Using the ball gives you full range of motion, unlike crunches on the floor.

- Sit on the ball with your feet resting on the floor and your back straight.
- Tighten your abdominal muscles and lean back. Keep your back straight!
- Return to the start position.
- Do a 10- to 15-rep set, rest for 1 minute, then repeat.

RESISTANCE BAND

Curl with a resistance band to work both the biceps and triceps muscles.

- Stand with both feet on the middle of the band and hold the handles with your palms facing outward.
- Bend your elbows to bring your palms toward your shoulders.

- Lower your forearms to the starting position.
- Do a 10- to 15-rep set, rest for 1 minute, then repeat.

DUMBBELLS

Doing flies with dumbbells works your shoulders and upper back.

- Holding a weight in each hand, with your palms toward your body, lean forward until your upper body is parallel to the floor and let your arms hang down. Keep your back straight.
- Keeping your arms straight, raise them out to the sides to shoulder level.
- Lower your arms to the starting position.
- Do a 10- to 15-rep set, rest for 1 minute, then repeat.

Side lunges, especially when done with weights, work your whole body.

- Stand with your feet hip-width apart with one weight in each hand, with your palms toward your body.
- Bend forward slightly at the waist and raise your arms to bring the dumbbells to shoulder level with your palms facing forward.
- Keeping your arms straight, do a side lunge to the left as you lower your right arm toward your left foot.
- Return to the center as you raise your right arm to its original position, then lunge to the right, bringing your left arm toward your right foot.
- Do a 10- to 15-rep set, rest for 1 minute, then repeat the set.

Torso twists work your abs, obliques, shoulders, and back.

- Stand with one weight in each hand, with your palms facing your body.
- Keep your hips facing forward.
- Curl the weights up so your hands are near your shoulders.
- Rotate your torso to the right, back to the center, and then to the left.
- Do a 10- to 15-rep set, rest for 1 minute, then repeat.

Alycia's workout is a great start for a home-based regimen. But make sure to keep having fun a top priority. Once you've successfully done this exercise program for 3 weeks, shake things up a bit. Get a fitness DVD or an exercise guide and try all the alternative moves the trainer suggests to keep challenging your body, keep increasing the intensity. The trick is to keep trying anything and everything you're interested in—don't feel like you have to stick with one thing. You don't want your muscles—or your brain—to get complacent.

Once you're on a steady streak with your exercise, you'll likely see a change in almost everything you do: You'll likely feel stronger, more energetic. You'll think more clearly, sleep better, be more focused in your work and home life. But inside your body, other positive developments can happen, many of them beyond your awareness. Those muscles you're building will start to become more sensitive to insulin, helping balance your blood sugar. Your testosterone level will increase, giving you more energy and enhancing your sex drive. Your blood level of the stress hormone cortisol will naturally start to level off and drop, helping you feel fully rested and relaxed. In other words, your hormone balance will start to right itself—an incredibly powerful total-body health shift that can impact your moods, your metabolism, even the rate at which your body ages. Not bad for a little workout, huh?

Now let's consider some 5-minute fixes that you can do to get your hormones back on an even keel, to create even more glorious time in your longer, happier, healthier life

Get a Handle on Your Hormones

You might read the title of this chapter and think, "I can skip reading this one—I'm a guy!" or "I don't have to worry about hormones for years yet." But hormones are not just a women's issue, and menopause certainly isn't the only time when hormones become unbalanced. Hormones are the secret agents of our interior world—we might not have a clue what they're doing, but these stealthy chemicals are at the center of the action, pulling strings and making things happen.

Hormones impact almost every single body process. In fact, no person—male or female—could even wake up in the morning or fall asleep at night without hormones doing the work they do.

The endocrine system is a dynamic communications network. Hormones are tireless little messengers that zoom out of their glands to deliver instructions either to other hormones or to the nervous system, reproductive system, kidneys, gut, liver, pancreas, and fat. The little busybodies help turn body processes on and off, as well as controlling their speed or intensity. They basically have a hand in everything from how much food you eat to how much sex you want to have to how intensely you react to stress—even how quickly or slowly your body ages.

Each of the hundreds of hormones in your body has at least one task. Some, like estrogen and testosterone, are heavy hitters, impacting dozens of aspects of health. Others may have just one or two jobs. But with scientists discovering new hormonal actions—and even new hormones—every day, endocrinology is a dynamic area of medicine that is truly at the forefront of science.

You may have heard talk in the news in the past few years about "endocrine disruptors"—things that are present in our daily lives and environment that interrupt the normal functioning of our hormones. While these news items may focus on toxic chemicals and plastics interrupting these important processes, excess fat can be one of the biggest endocrine disruptors that hangs on our bodies 24/7.

Excess fat is the number one risk factor for developing one of the most debilitating hormonal imbalances, diabetes. The lifetime risk of diabetes among people in the United States is now 30 to 40 percent—not coincidentally, almost the same percentage of people who are obese. The most common form of diabetes, type 2, happens when our bodies can no longer properly process or maybe even produce the hormone insulin to manage our blood sugar effectively. Diabetes in adulthood raises our risks for almost every other chronic illness, especially heart disease. Indeed, diabetes raises the risk of heart attack by as much as having had a previous heart attack does. The average person who develops diabetes will have his life shortened by a tragic 13 years.

The spread of diabetes is a crisis in our country, but it is one that we can begin to seriously remedy in the next 5 minutes. No kidding. If we take care of the blood's insulin balance, we will automatically be taking care of most of our other metabolic hormones, so we'll focus most of our 5-minute fixes in that arena. But let's first learn about the endocrine system that insulin balance is such a huge part of—and then we'll learn some very small, manageable steps that we can take to protect it right away.

Fix It in 5
Keep Hormones on an Even Keel

1. Eat lean protein with every meal.
2. Sleep for 7 to 8 hours a night.
3. Avoid exposure to industrial pollutants and other toxic chemicals.
4. Maintain a healthy weight.
5. Exercise for at least 30 minutes a day.

A 5-Minute Tour of Your Endocrine System

Hormones help regulate almost everything in our bodies—our moods, rate of growth, sexual prowess, even the speed of our metabolism—after being produced in a system of glands located throughout the body. Once they are dispatched from those glands, hormones set out to deliver instructions to various organs and cells in the body. The mastermind behind this messaging system is the hypothalamus, a gland in the lower part of the brain. The hypothalamus is like the control room, receiving messages from other body systems and directing the pituitary gland, which sits just below the hypothalamus, to create and dispatch other hormones. Check out some of the amazing functions each little gland and its hormones are capable of.

Pituitary Gland. This gland is the right-hand man to the hypothalamus, directing lots of hormonal traffic. The pituitary kicks off many hormonal "cascades" in the body, sending out signal hormones that then kick other hormones into action. The many hormones the pituitary produces include:

- Human growth hormone, which stimulates the growth of bones and tissues and is often called "the elixir of youth" for its power to keep muscles strong and skin smooth
- Prolactin, a hormone that activates milk production in breastfeeding women
- Thyrotropin, which stimulates the thyroid gland (see below)
- Corticotropin, which triggers hormone production in the adrenal gland (see next page)
- Endorphins, feel-good hormones produced when you exercise
- Oxytocin, the fun hormone that helps you have an orgasm, fall in love, and feed a baby—not to mention triggers the contractions that let you have that baby

Pineal Gland. This teeny gland is nestled right between the two hemispheres of the brain, where it secretes melatonin, the hormone that regulates sleep and controls our whole wake–sleep cycle.

Thyroid Gland. This gland sits right below the Adam's apple. This baby takes in iodine from your diet and turns it into thyroxine (T4) or triiodothyronine (T3), the hormones that control metabolism, the rate at which we turn oxygen and calories into energy. Every cell in our bodies relies upon thyroid hormones to help regulate that metabolism, so obviously they're pretty critical! Thyroid hormones also determine the rate of kids' bone growth. Another hormone produced in the thyroid, calcitonin, acts to reduce calcium while opposing the action of parathyroid hormone, which tends to raise blood calcium. The calcium floating around in our bloodstream is closely kept within a normal range of 8 to 10 mg/dL. If blood calcium falls rapidly below or above this range, the heart stops beating or can develop an unstable rhythm leading to death.

Parathyroid Glands. These are four small glands hidden behind the thyroid, and their main job is to raise blood calcium through the action of parathyroid hormone (PTH). In addition to the impact of calcium on the heart, extremely low or high blood calcium can cause seizures or coma. Interestingly, even in people with severe osteoporosis, a calcium-deficient disease, serum calcium is kept normal by PTH. If blood calcium falls, PTH simply chips more calcium out of your bones. Your body will literally eat up your skeleton to keep your blood calcium from dropping.

Adrenal Glands. We've got two of these, a matched set that sit on top of each kidney. The adrenals are important to the stress response—how we experience it and how our bodies react to it. Cortisol and catecholamines (epinephrine and norepinephrine) are all stress hormones that help energize us to get the job done. A little release of stress hormones keeps things interesting—but too much can eventually be deadly. Another adrenal hormone, aldosterone, regulates blood pressure and salt and water balance in the body. Dehydroepiandrosterone (DHEA) and testosterone are also produced by the adrenal gland.

Pancreas. This biggie is all about keeping the body fueled with a steady source of energy. If we have too little blood sugar, the pancreas releases glucagon to raise it; if we have too much, it releases insulin to lower it. When the pancreas is bugged over and over to release insulin to accommodate high blood sugar caused by overeating, it can start to shut down—and we get type 2 diabetes.

Ovaries. Along with producing the eggs that created us all, the ovaries produce estrogen and progesterone. Estrogen is best known for bringing us such changes as puberty and pregnancy, and it also has dozens of actions that keep a woman's body healthy and strong. When a woman

I've heard a lot about type 2 diabetes—but how will I know if my child has type 1 diabetes? What are the signs? How long should I wait before calling my doctor?

A child with type 1 diabetes will become seriously ill, usually with vomiting and an altered state of consciousness. This happens because when type 1 diabetes occurs, the body is making little or no insulin, so the blood sugar doesn't get escorted into the cells and, instead, remains in the bloodstream—and the body can't get the sugar where it needs it. Any sign of changes in level of consciousness, with or without vomiting, or drinking or urinating excessively might mean high blood sugar and requires urgent care. Call your pediatrician first—but if you can't reach him or her, head to the ER.

—*Charles I. Shubin, MD, director of pediatrics,*
Mercy FamilyCare, a division of Family Health Centers of Baltimore

loses all estrogen at menopause, this can lead to increased risk of heart disease, osteoporosis, and Alzheimer's disease. Progesterone is estrogen's lesser-known but equally powerful sister that helps regulate the menstrual cycle and is especially active during pregnancy. Other cells in the ovaries produce 50 percent of a woman's testosterone (the remainder comes from the adrenal glands). While women have much lower amounts of testosterone than men have, it's still important in maintaining their energy, sex drive, and muscle tone.

Testes. These low-rider glands are home to the "male" sex hormones, like testosterone, that bring on puberty and control sexual function as well as doing fun things like keeping our thinking sharp, making us randy, and helping us build strong muscles. All you guys may think that testosterone is only about sex, but it's also very important in protecting you against heart disease because it supports the heart muscle, which is constantly pumping 24/7.

Keep Insulin on an Even Keel

As we mentioned earlier, by far the biggest preventable threat to health is type 2 diabetes. According to the CDC, if current trends continue, 1 in 3 Americans will develop diabetes sometime in their lifetime, and if you have diabetes, you will lose, on average, 10 to 15 years of life. Both type 1 and type 2 diabetes affect blood sugar regulation, but while type 1 is an unfortunate twist of fate, the other is almost entirely preventable.

RED FLAG: PREDIABETES AND DIABETES

Millions of Americans have type 2 diabetes, but don't know it. Scarily, many more have prediabetes, which is slightly higher than normal blood sugar levels that mean your odds of developing full-blown diabetes are dramatically higher. If you have prediabetes, making healthy lifestyle changes can markedly lower your risk for developing the disease itself.

Many people with prediabetes have no symptoms. However, there may be warning signs that are easy to overlook. Here's how to catch them.

- Ask your doctor about having a fasting blood sugar check if you have risk factors for prediabetes or diabetes. That's you if you're over age 45 or if you're overweight and any of these are true: you have an inactive lifestyle, high blood pressure, low levels of "good" HDL cholesterol, or a family history of diabetes (in a parent, brother, or sister), or if you are African American, Asian American, Hispanic, Native American, or Pacific Islander.

- Watch for prediabetes red flags. These include darkened skin in body folds, such as on the sides of the neck, under the arms, and in the groin, or on the elbows, knees, or knuckles.

- Check for diabetes warning signs. Call your doctor right away for an appointment if you have unusual fatigue, excessive thirst and/or hunger, frequent urination, unexpected weight loss, cuts and bruises that are slow to heal, tingling or numbness in your hands or feet, or infections of the skin, gums, or bladder that keep returning. (You could also have type 2 diabetes without having any symptoms, so if you notice one of these, consider it a gift—and definitely get checked out.)

Type 1 diabetes is an autoimmune disease that usually shows up in childhood or early adolescence. The immune system mistakenly attacks pancreatic cells making insulin, and with the loss of these cells, you develop type 1 diabetes. Type 1 diabetes requires daily insulin injections or delivery by an infusion pump attached to a needle catheter, which must be worn continuously. For the person with type 1 diabetes, life is filled with constant calculations of how much sugar is in the blood, how much energy has been expended, and how much insulin is needed. Living with type 1 requires constant vigilance; otherwise, it can lead to very serious complications, including kidney failure, blindness, amputation, nerve damage, stroke—and even death. Medicine has advanced markedly in the past few decades, however, and instruments such as automatic insulin pumps now allow at least a degree of freedom. With close monitoring, a person with type 1 diabetes can enjoy a healthier life than was possible even 10 years ago.

Another type of diabetes, type 2, is preventable. It starts when your normal hormonal process is taxed to its limits. The process goes like this: You eat some food. The food is digested and broken down into glucose (aka sugar), which is then released into the bloodstream. Your pancreas responds to this elevated glucose level and pumps out some insulin, which joins up with the glucose molecules and shuttles them from the blood vessels to the cells of the body to be used as energy.

When you are very overweight, your pancreas may gradually stop making insulin or your body's cells may lose their ability to recognize it, a condition called insulin resistance. The glucose can't get into your cells and instead builds up in the blood. Not only does glucose cause harm when it builds up in the bloodstream, it also doesn't give your cells what they need for their basic functions. Your pancreas, sensing all of this sugar in your blood, produces more and more insulin to bind with it, but eventually it maxes out and shuts down.

High glucose levels over the long term can damage your kidneys, eyes, and heart as well as increase your risk of heart attack and stroke. If left unchecked, high blood sugar gradually destroys blood vessels, nerves, and organs.

Fighting Fat, the Forgotten Gland

Unfortunately, when we have insulin resistance, our bodies tend to store extra weight right where we shouldn't have it: around our waists.

For decades, researchers believed our fat was just . . . there. They thought it was blobs of inert jelly, just hanging out, making our pants tighter. But in recent decades, endocrine researchers have discovered that fat, especially visceral (belly) fat, is anything but static.

Our fat cells actually produce several hormones, one of which can be beneficial: leptin. When everything works the way it should, leptin gets released when we eat and alerts the brain to turn off the appetite signal, making us feel satiated after a meal.

Unfortunately, having excess fat throws off leptin production, causing our cells to develop leptin resistance in the same way that they develop insulin resistance. Once we shed a few pounds and shrink some of those belly fat cells, they stop producing so much leptin and the system functions normally again. Studies have shown that healthy centenarians have leptin levels very similar to the levels of much younger adults, which suggests that optimizing leptin levels may be one of the many keys to staying healthy well into our older years.

Another hormone associated with the stomach—but actually produced in the gut, or intestines—is ghrelin, a true hunger hormone. Ghrelin is what makes our mouths water at the smell—or even the thought!—of our favorite foods. At lunchtime, ghrelin reminds us that it's time to eat by making its way to the hypothalamus to trigger the release of neuropeptide Y, a powerful neurochemical that drives appetite. Ghrelin's actions get stronger the more we overeat. If we have a habit of snacking throughout the day, our levels of this hormone rise more often and neuropeptide Y becomes an all-powerful master that is very difficult to ignore.

Protect Your Energy Flow

We can exert some control over the hormones related to our digestion, but we have less of a say about some of our other hormones—including those produced by the thyroid. Most of us probably never give a thought to the thyroid. It just sucks that iodine out of food, makes its thyroid hormones, helps our bodies convert energy, and that's that. But sometimes, due mostly to heredity, pregnancy, aging—and, increasingly, environmental factors—the thyroid can get out of whack.

If the thyroid starts to create too many hormones, you develop hyperthyroidism—you'll lose weight, sweat excessively, and often develop a swelling in the neck called a goiter. But what's more common as we age is hypothyroidism, when the levels of the thyroid hormones are low. Then, we tend to have extremely low energy levels and may start gaining weight. Many women encounter low thyroid function after they give birth, but those changes often dissipate as the months go by (low thyroid function can contribute to postpartum depression, so see your doctor if it's severe or lasts several weeks). Many diseases and conditions can contribute to thyroid malfunction, though, so it's important that your doctor checks your thyroid hormone levels when you have your annual blood work done.

Another source of thyroid issues can be chronic stress, which can really do a number on the entire endocrine system. When we overtax our adrenals on an ongoing basis, getting worked up over deadlines or fights with family, we overproduce the stress hormones epinephrine, norepinephrine, and cortisol. Of these, cortisol is clearly the most damaging—it makes us eat more (especially fats and sweets), converts healthy hip fat into toxic belly fat, suppresses the

DOCTOR, DOCTOR, GIMME THE NEWS: PAINKILLERS MAY REDUCE CANCER RISKS

A study published in *Cancer Epidemiology, Biomarkers and Prevention* examined the use of aspirin, nonsteroidal anti-inflammatory drugs (NSAIDs), and acetaminophen among 740 postmenopausal women and found that using these painkillers lowered their levels of estradiol, a form of estrogen, by 10.5 percent—a drop that just might help prevent certain cancers.

The painkillers have chemicals that mimic the body's natural aromatase, an enzyme that helps convert androgens to estrogens. By decreasing the action of prostaglandins (a type of hormone associated with inflammation and cell growth), aspirin and other painkillers may also decrease the action of aromatase, which in turn decreases estrogen. Lower estrogen levels after menopause have been linked to reduced risks of breast and ovarian cancer. The study's author, Margaret A. Gates, ScD, a research fellow at Brigham and Women's Hospital's Channing Laboratory in Boston, says additional research is still needed to confirm the association between use of analgesics and estrogen levels, and to determine whether this translates into a lower risk of breast or ovarian cancer. But future randomized trials looking at aspirin, non-aspirin NSAID, and acetaminophen use and changes in hormone levels should help to confirm any link between the drugs and estrogen levels and to figure out the most effective doses.

immune system, and generally raises our risk of heart disease. Too much cortisol can prevent our brains from creating new memories or being able to access old ones.

In general terms, men and women tend to deal with stress differently, and both styles have their pros and cons. Adrenaline can be positive (when running away from danger, for example), but if it's activated for a long time it can have adverse effects on your health. Do positive things to decrease your stress, such as getting massages or regular exercise.

Stay Sexy and Strong

The hormones produced in the ovaries ebb and flow depending on a woman's reproductive life stage, and it's that careful balance between estrogen, progesterone, and a bit of the androgens that keeps things interesting from your very first period to the last (and all those many, many monthly cycles in between).

As time marches on, however, those sex hormones wane, and whether you're ready for them or not, the effects can be dramatic. In menopause, when all the eggs have been used up, the body acknowledges that the time for having babies is over. This process actually begins in your late thirties, as the ovaries start making less estrogen and progesterone and fewer healthy eggs are available for possible fertilization, making it more difficult to get pregnant than it was when you were younger. As the hormonal decline progresses into your forties, you may notice a change in your periods and, eventually, periods stop altogether. Some women find the transition to menopause to be a challenge, first being troubled by the hot flashes, night sweats, and weight gain and later having increased risks of heart disease, osteoporosis, and Alzheimer's disease. Most women still produce small amounts of testosterone, but without adequate estrogen, it can lead to facial whiskers, loss of scalp hair, acne, and a deepening of the voice commonly seen in older women. While there's still controversy about taking female hormones, you don't have to passively stand by and watch your body fall apart. Seek out an endocrinologist, gynecologist, or other knowledgeable physician to advise you on whether hormone therapy is right for you.

One

Hormone, 16 Benefits
Vitamin D

Vitamin D might not sound like a hormone, but it acts like one in the body, traveling throughout the system and turning on and off dozens of body processes in the brain, heart, skin, and several glands. Vitamin D receptors are also involved in regulating the immune system and helping to manage the response to infection and inflammation. A huge wave of studies about vitamin D that have appeared over the past few years have underscored how important this nutrient is—and how lacking we've been in it for far too long. More than 50 percent of all adults and maybe as many as 70 percent of children have lower levels of vitamin D than they should, and as many as 10 percent may be highly deficient.

And while it would be ideal to be able to get enough vitamin D from our food, our bodies are much more efficient at making our own vitamin D if we get enough sunlight. If we get 20 to 30 minutes of summer sun, our skin will produce as much as 10,000 IU of vitamin D—50 times more than the US government's recommendation of 200 IU per day. (To put that in perspective, you'd have to drink 100 glasses of milk to get that much from your diet.) And while much controversy swirls around how much to take as a supplement, which kind of supplement is best, and how much is too much, you should keep this in mind: It is virtually impossible to overdose on vitamin D from any food source or from the sun. In one study of more than

Ladies, you may be relieved to know that you are not alone: Yes, men can go through a "male menopause," too. But it's not quite the same. While 100 percent of women go through menopause, even when men experience a decline in testosterone, it rarely drops to zero. While it's not common, there have been reported cases in the literature of healthy men in their nineties achieving paternity. Lucky guys!

A more typical pattern for an aging man is for testosterone levels to decline in about 30 percent of men beginning in their forties and fifties. The lower levels of testosterone can

500,000 people from 10 European countries, the higher the level of vitamin D in their blood, the lower their risk of colon cancer. Researchers believe the protective effect of the higher vitamin D levels were associated with sun exposure.

Now, please—we're not advocating that you sit out and bake in the sun. But certainly try to get those good 20 to 30 minutes of unobstructed sunlight every day. If you're an officeworker, head outside the womb of the office building at noon and take a walk in the sun for the second half of your lunch hour. Always wear sunscreen on your face, and even wear a hat—no sun damage for you! But roll up your sleeves and make sure you can feel the sun's warmth on your skin—it feels good, and it's good for you. Consider what science suggests that vitamin D can do:

1. Build strong bones
2. Prevent osteoporosis
3. Reduce the rate of asthma
4. Decrease the risk of developing multiple sclerosis
5. Reduce physical disability and cognitive impairment in people with multiple sclerosis
6. Cut breast, colon, and prostate cancer risk
7. Decrease the risk of heart attack and stroke
8. Reduce blood pressure
9. Enhance immunity
10. Decrease the risk of type 1 diabetes
11. Help enhance insulin sensitivity and decrease insulin resistance
12. Help prevent diabetes
13. Help maintain a healthy weight
14. Reduce depression
15. Reduce the risk of developing and relieve the symptoms of autism
16. Prevent development of autoimmune disorders like rheumatoid arthritis and inflammatory bowel disease

impact erectile function, libido, and take away that natural advantage for muscle power that they've enjoyed throughout their lives. Remember low testosterone can also contribute to increased risks of heart disease because your heart muscle needs to pump 24/7. If levels become truly deficient, seek out an endocrinologist or other knowledgeable physician to evaluate the cause of your low testosterone and to advise you on your options for therapy. There are some causes of low testosterone that are reversible, so don't be satisfied with just being put on testosterone treatment.

5-Minute Fixes

for a Lifetime of Hormonal Health

The thing about hormones is, there's only so much you can do to impact each individual hormone directly—i.e., not much. Because the endocrine system is so interconnected, any attempt you make to unnaturally "boost" one may just result in another getting out of whack. It's better to let the body regulate its own hormones while we do everything we can to take care of ourselves in more general ways: Sleep more. Eat less. Chill out. Have fun. Sounds doable, right? Let's consider a few fun ways to get there.

RED FLAG: METABOLIC SYNDROME

Metabolic syndrome *looks* like a collection of small and unrelated health problems. But don't ignore them. If you have metabolic syndrome, your cells resist insulin—the hormone that tells your body to absorb blood sugar. This raises your risk for developing diabetes fivefold and can double your odds for heart disease. A study of nearly 5,000 women published in the *Archives of Neurology* found that developing metabolic syndrome resulted in a 23 percent increase in the risk of developing cognitive impairment.

But losing weight; eating a healthy diet packed with fruits, vegetables, whole grains, and lean protein; and exercising regularly can all help to reverse it.

While metabolic syndrome shares some characteristics of prediabetes, you officially have metabolic syndrome if you have three or more of these red flags:

- A waist measurement of 40 inches or more for men, 35 inches or more for women
- Triglyceride levels of 150 milligrams per deciliter (mg/dL) or above, or you are taking medication for high triglycerides
- An HDL, or "good," cholesterol level of below 40 mg/dL for men and below 50 mg/dL for women, or you are taking medication to raise low HDL levels
- Blood pressure of 130/85 mmHg or above, or you are taking medication for high blood pressure
- A fasting blood sugar level of 100 mg/dL or above, or you are taking medication for high blood sugar

---

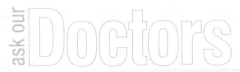

My doctor just told me I have prediabetes, and I'm scared to death. What do I do now?

If you want to reduce their risk for diabetes, you need to maintain a healthy weight—that's it. The proven strength of this recommendation is tremendous. You get more results from this than any drug therapy—it's very powerful. Your body benefits metabolically from just a small amount of weight loss. So don't focus on achieving what would be considered "normal" weight—just move in the direction of weight loss and shoot for 5 to 10 percent of body weight loss.

Brisk walking also benefits insulin resistance, even in moderate amounts. You should aim for 20 to 30 minutes of walking over the course of the day. Taking stairs instead of the elevator can make a difference, even just one flight, or parking your car far from the grocery store and walking a little more. Preventing type 2 diabetes is a lifestyle issue: Developing habits around how you go through your day-to-day life is what matters.

—Elizabeth Mayer-Davis, MSPH, PhD, RD, president-elect,
health care and education, American Diabetes Association

Try to stay out of the pharmacy. If you're edging ever closer to diabetes, it might be tempting to control your blood sugar with drugs. Doctors often reach for their prescription pads because they assume that patients will not follow a strict diet and exercise program. Have a serious talk with your doctor about changing your lifestyle and he or she will likely give you a few more months to get your blood sugar under control before starting you on medication, which could be a good thing because no medicine has been proven to be nearly as effective as diet and exercise for preventing or reversing diabetes. In fact, large-scale studies have found that people with prediabetes can prevent diabetes and reverse the course of their disease simply by reducing fat and calories and walking for 30 minutes a day, 5 days a week. Research has shown that people who lost just 5 to 7 percent of their weight cut their risk of developing diabetes by nearly 60 percent—that was twice as effective as metformin, the most widely prescribed antidiabetes drug, which cut the risk by 31 percent. Some recent large-scale studies in people with diabetes have produced conflicting results about the effects of aggressively lowering blood sugar and of managing heart disease risk by reducing blood pressure—and none of it is that promising. Bottom line, stick with what research has proven works best—exercising more and losing weight—and do everything you can to resist the urge to run to the bottle. Talk to your doctor about giving you extra time to make changes with lifestyle strategies, and work your hardest to avoid drugs. **Time spent:** less time at the pharmacy, more time out walking the dog (30 minutes a day)

Swap white rice for brown. Research presented at an American Heart Association conference in San Francisco in March 2010 found a direct connection between the type of rice consumed and diabetes risk. By studying roughly 200,000 people, the researchers determined that those who ate five or more servings of white rice a week were 17 percent more likely to develop diabetes than people who ate less than one serving a month. Meanwhile, those who ate two or more servings of brown rice per week were 11 percent less likely to develop diabetes than those who ate less than one serving a month.

With 2 grams of fiber and just more than 100 calories per half cup, brown rice takes a bit longer to cook—45 minutes versus 15 to 20 minutes for white rice. Because of the longer cooking time, you might want to make extra, which you can store for up to a week in the fridge (6 months in the freezer). Start your transition from white rice with quick-cooking brown rice before moving over to regular brown rice. Once you get used to it, the nutty flavor can be a welcome change from bland white rice. **Time spent:** 45 minutes once a week versus 15 minutes several times a week

Take some *natural* vitamin E. One review published in the journal *Experimental Gerontology* found that healthy centenarians, people who have lived to age 100 with vitality and

My daughter is only 8 and she's starting
to get breasts! What's going on?

Dr. Jim says . . .

I share your concern—I'm seeing this problem increasingly in my practice. Many girls are developing and getting their periods earlier than ever. We're not sure exactly why this happens in every case, but we do know that girls who gain weight the fastest between 36 months of age and first grade tend to have a higher risk, as do those who have a higher BMI (over the 85th percentile) when they're 36 months old—so childhood obesity is definitely a factor. What also worries me are the increased amounts of exogenous estrogens in our environment from some of the thousands of unregulated chemicals such as phthalates, which are found in lotions and shampoos (usually masquerading in ingredient lists as "fragrance"). They were recently found by researchers at Mount Sinai to be associated with earlier breast and pubic hair development. Also troubling is bisphenol A (BPA), a type of plastic that has been used in baby bottles as well as many other products for years, way before the government or industry started to acknowledge how dangerous it might be. We now know that even small exposures to BPA—which is everywhere, from the lining of cans of food to the receipts we get at the gas pump—can increase estrogenic effects in the body. Five percent of all the BPA made is used in products that directly touch food, and pesticides and hormones in that food may also be contributing their own estrogenic effects.

While no one wants his or her little girl to grow up too fast, there are dire health risks here as well. Early menstruation is also a risk factor for breast cancer, because their little bodies seem to have higher levels of estrogen. Do what you can to make sure your daughter gets plenty of exercise to prevent obesity—1 hour of vigorous running, playing, jumping, climbing trees every day!—and plenty of fresh (not canned) organic fruits, vegetables, and lean proteins. It's not a bad idea for you, too!

Doctors

I've heard so much about bioidentical
hormones. Can you tell me—are they safer
than regular hormone replacement therapy?

Indeed, much confusion surrounds hormone therapy for women. It all started when the Women's Health Initiative (WHI), published in 2002, showed Prempro (the most commonly prescribed hormone therapy in the United States, a combination of synthetic horse estrogen and synthetic progestin taken by mouth) caused increased heart attacks, strokes, and breast cancer. The study also found that Premarin, a synthetic horse estrogen–only formulation delivered orally, offered no protection against heart disease.

These results were followed by mass panic, and millions of women were abruptly taken off all female hormones or stopped them on their own. The FDA required all pharmaceutical companies making estrogen to include warnings about its risks on their product information, based on the WHI findings. So despite offering a different product, companies making pharmaceutical topical estradiol were forced by the FDA to include the WHI risks on their product information. Not surprisingly, women became very distrustful and fearful of all pharmaceutical hormones.

Not long thereafter, there were many high-profile endorsements for compounded bioidentical hormones, and women flocked to compounding pharmacies. Compounding pharmacists can provide a valuable service, especially for patients with allergies to pharmaceuticals or for products no longer commercially available. But compounding pharmacists have never been required to issue any warning labels on their products, so naturally women assumed compounded bioidenticals had no risks—which is certainly not the case. It is important for women to understand that any estrogen carries risks, but the risks from bioidentical topical estrogen are fewer than the risks from Premarin and Prempro.

By definition, a bioidentical hormone is simply a product identical to the molecular structure of the naturally occurring hormones that exist in a woman's body. All bioidentical hormones, whether pharmaceutical or compounded, are made from plant estrogens, which are synthesized in the labora-

mobility, are more likely to have dramatically lower rates of insulin resistance than those who are much younger than them. In fact, they had the lowest rates of any of the other age groups studied, from age 26 up to 90. The researchers believe this backs up a theory that

tory to be identical to human estradiol. (After all, we are not geraniums! So we need to modify plant estrogens.) Topical estrogens include patches, creams, and gels of estradiol, and may help reduce the risk of weight gain (especially around the middle), sexual dysfunction, heart disease, strokes, gallstones, and migraines.

The critical difference between pharmaceutical and compounded bioidentical hormones is that pharmaceutical companies have to follow stricter manufacturing standards and ensure quality control of their products. Celebrities endorsing proprietary compounded hormones make outlandish claims despite the fact there has never been any published clinical trial on compounded bioidentical hormones—any published study quoted was conducted using pharmaceutical topical estradiol products. (Note: The improved safety of topical over oral pharmaceutical bioidentical hormones has been shown in hundreds of publications from mainstream medical journals.)

In my practice, I have prescribed both compounded and pharmaceutical bioidentical products. I always prefer pharmaceutical hormone products because they provide better, more consistent results. (It's very common for me to see an initial patient who comes in on compounded hormone products from another physician and their blood estradiol is zero!) I use compounded hormone products primarily in patients with special allergies or for bioidentical products that are not commercially available, but they have to be closely monitored as I do with all hormone therapy.

Bottom line? With correct monitoring of blood levels, pharmaceutical and compounded bioidentical hormones are safer than the synthetic estrogen products used in WHI. But all women are individuals. Talk to your doctor about which works best for you. And if you want to check out bioidentical hormones, please be sure you see a board-certified endocrinologist or gynecologist. Enter your doctor's name at www.abim.org/services/verify-a-physician.aspx to check their board certification credentials, or go to the Hormone Foundation's Web site (www.hormone.org) to find an endocrinologist or gynecologist near you.

—**Marina Johnson, MD, FACE,** *founder and medical director of the Institute of Endocrinology and Preventive Medicine in the Dallas–Fort Worth Metroplex and author of* Outliving Your Ovaries

those who live beyond 100 have much greater sensitivity to and efficient use of insulin than any other group.

The same review found that these healthy centenarians were also much more likely to have lower levels of oxidative stress and higher circulating levels of vitamin E. Oxidative stress may increase the risk of heart disease, and vice versa—it's a vicious circle. Does vitamin E help manage that? Scientists are not entirely sure, but we say it might be worth a try. Another National Institutes of Health–funded study published in the *New England Journal of Medicine* found that daily vitamin E supplementation may help improve the livers of people struggling with nonalcoholic steatohepatitis (NASH), a condition common in people with diabetes. After taking 800 IU of vitamin E in its natural form daily, the livers of 43 percent of the people with NASH showed significant improvement, compared with only 19 percent of those who received a placebo. Some studies have suggested that supplemental vitamin E improves insulin action and glucose disposal in not only people with type 2 diabetes, but also in nondiabetics. Just be sure to get natural vitamin E—d-alpha tocopherol, not dl-alpha tocopherol. It's a bit more expensive, but lower-quality synthetic vitamin E has been associated with risks. You can also get vitamin E from almonds—a great source—sunflower seeds or oil, hazelnuts, and avocados. **Time spent:** 15 seconds every morning to take that capsule or grab those nuts

Throw out any fast food coupons in the house—now! Fast food is cheap, though its effects on our health could cost us in the long run. But when researchers from the University of North Carolina at Chapel Hill followed 5,000 people over 20 years, they found that as prices of fast food and soda went up, consumption went down. For example, when costs went up 1 percent, people consumed 7.1 fewer calories from soda and 11.5 percent fewer calories from pizza a day, translating to roughly 56 fewer calories a day and potentially 3 to 4 pounds of weight loss each year! They also had a lower risk of diabetes thanks to their lower fasting levels of insulin. Impose your own fast food tax by removing the temptation to get a "deal" on fast food—it's never worth the price. **Time spent:** 2 minutes to round up your coupon folder and toss them all!

Go ahead, have the cheese omelette. A recent study from the University of Alabama in Tuscaloosa found that animals fed higher-fat meals for breakfast had healthier levels of

I'm really afraid that my husband is not interested in having sex anymore. He can get an erection—but it's just so rare that he even asks for sex. What's going on? Is his testosterone level falling?

This is a frequent concern for couples, especially as they get into midlife. If they have a good relationship with a healthy sex life and suddenly things start to dwindle, it's understandable to be concerned. When they can't perform sexually, some men will react by simply avoiding sex for fear of failure. It's important to rule out major stress or illness, which can make anyone lose interest in sex. However, if he has symptoms of night sweats, poor sleep, or weight gain around the middle, please encourage him to be screened with a total and free testosterone. If it's low, it's important to undergo a diagnostic evaluation to determine the cause of the low testosterone, especially because some cases are reversible. For example, a serious condition like sleep apnea can be a common cause of low testosterone; I have seen many instances where treatment of the sleep apnea completely normalized testosterone levels.

—Marina Johnson, MD, FACE

metabolic hormones than those who ate breakfasts higher in carbohydrates. Researchers believe that by eating fat soon after awakening, the body's metabolism was efficiently turned on, which also allowed the animal to get the maximum benefit from other types of foods eaten later in the day. In contrast, the animals who were fed more carbs upon awakening actually processed food differently all day long, and their bodies seemed to absorb the carbs more readily than other nutrients. At the end of the study, the carb-breakfast animals had gained weight and body fat, had developed glucose intolerance, and were developing other signs of metabolic syndrome.

The researchers said that in order for humans to make this pattern work for them, they should eat a lower-calorie meal for dinner. If you can do that, we say enjoy the full-fat cheese omelette, guilt-free, every so often—but, as a rule, on most days, stuff that omelette with healthier sources of fat, like the omega-3s in smoked salmon or organic breakfast sausage from your local farmer's market. Also choose organic eggs that are high in omega-3s and throw in some healthy veggies. **Time spent:** just a bit more time to whip up an omelette—2 minutes—than to toast up a bagel

Have a laugh—an intense one. While the negative stress of chronic overwork and worry can do a number on our stress hormones, we do have ways to tap into our positive, joyful hormones. The body has a very well-developed system in place to relieve stress through positive emotions—but sometimes we just have to give it a kick start. Researchers at the Loma Linda University School of Medicine in California have found that intense laughter helps to optimize many of the body's functions. For example, they've shown that laughter increases the production and activity of antibodies and protective T cells in the immune system. They've even shown that regular intense laughter can affect the body almost like physical exercise, lowering blood pressure, decreasing stress hormones, increasing "good" cholesterol, and decreasing "bad."

Pick a night every week to watch something funny—a comedy show, some goofy YouTube videos, or a DVD from your favorite comedian. If you're a Netflix member, do some digging in its library of comedies and put a favorite comedian's latest into every third spot on your queue, so you always have some good chuckles coming your way. Or if you have a friend who always makes you laugh, plan to have dinner and drinks with him or her at least once a month. Studies have shown that simply looking forward to seeing a funny movie or laughing with friends can measurably lower your stress hormone levels. **Time spent:** get in at least an hour of hard-core laughing a week, even if it's just 10 minutes a day of getting tickled by your toddler or your partner

Schedule that hormone screen. If you're packing a few more pounds than you need and you've never had an endocrine assay, get one now. Gaining as little as 11 to 18 pounds doubles your chance of developing type 2 diabetes. In some respects, the months and years before diabetes is diagnosed are the most dangerous. Before you are even aware of the destructive forces at work in your body, you could be doing long-term damage to vital organs. In a study funded by the Centers for Disease Control and Prevention, researchers looked at the lab tests of 8,200 Americans and found that 42 percent of the people with undiagnosed diabetes had chronic kidney disease—similar to the 40 percent rate in those with diagnosed diabetes—and 18 percent of the subjects with prediabetes had it. Among people who had neither diabetes nor prediabetes, the rate of chronic kidney disease was about 11 percent.

When you get tested for diabetes, be sure to ask for a hemoglobin A1c test in addition to the traditional blood sugar testing. This newer blood test does a better job of predicting the risk of heart disease and stroke than the old fasting blood sugar test does. The hemoglobin A1c, or glycated hemoglobin, test measures average blood sugar levels over the past few months. Check with your doctor's office to see what tests your health insurance will cover.
Time spent: 5 minutes to schedule a test

Open up a test kitchen. Both cinnamon and apple cider vinegar have been shown to reduce blood sugar—cinnamon alone by anywhere from 18 to 29 percent—but the effect can be short-lived. One of the best things about these two items in combination, however, is how they can help you feel satisfied after a meal.

If you like experimenting in the kitchen, see if you can come up with any recipes that use both of these ingredients. Try mixing apple cider vinegar and cinnamon into a dressing to pour over cabbage or mix with apples for a tangy fruit salad. Otherwise, consider using vinegar (any type) as a "sprinkle" on high-carb foods such as potatoes. Some evidence suggests that fermented foods like vinegar contain acetic acid, which lowers blood sugar by helping move excess glucose to the liver for storage. While you're at it, throw a dash of cinnamon in everything you can stand it in—oatmeal, pancakes, coffee, tea, chili, spaghetti sauce, soup. While neither product will banish high blood sugar all by itself, both just may help you manage your cravings until the next meal. **Time spent:** 1 minute to sprinkle vinegar or cinnamon (or both) over your plate or cup

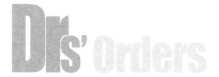

Drs' Orders
for Hormone Health:
Avoid Toxic Foods and Chemicals
and Endocrine Disruptors

We want to take a moment here to really stress the importance of getting toxins out of our lives—they are truly messing with our hormonal balance.

Now, just take a step back and consider all the different ways that toxins enter our lives. It's not just in the obvious ways—weed killers on our lawns, chlorine bleach in our washing machines, paint thinners in our garages. These endocrine-disrupting chemicals are in and on almost everything that touches our bodies and goes in our mouths. Let's just give one small example, the tip of the tip of the iceberg.

You know those oh-so-helpful nonstick pans we've been heating up and using to cook our food for more than 50 years? A study published in the peer-reviewed journal *Environmental Health Perspectives* recently linked the perfluorooctanoic acid (PFOA) that's used to make the nonstick coating with thyroid disease. The people with the highest (top 25th percentile) concentrations of PFOA in the blood were more than twice as likely to be on medication for thyroid disease as people with the lowest concentrations (the bottom 50th percentile). While this was the first human study to establish a link, animal studies have shown similar compounds may also disrupt thyroid hormones in the blood or change the way they're metabolized in the liver. Other studies have found that PFOA causes birth defects; increases cancer rates; and causes changes in the immune system, liver function, and blood lipid levels in animals—will we soon learn they do in people, too?

Now consider that PFOA is found in microwave popcorn bags, stain-resistant carpets, waterproof clothing, house dust, and industrial waste—even our drinking water—even though a concerted effort is underway to limit its use.

Thankfully, the EPA has decreed that PFOAs cannot be used in making pans beginning in 2015. But these chemicals can take 10 years or more to leave the body—and with the amount of PFOA floating around in the world, we could be exposed to it for many decades to come.

Okay, here's the really scary part: Multiply that potential effect by the *thousands* of chemicals found in our environment and even the sometimes reticent Environmental Protection Agency starts to get a little overwhelmed: "It is difficult to make generalizations about the effects of chemicals and chemical usage, not only because there are thousands of chemicals, but also because individual chemicals have unique ways of being absorbed and handled by living organisms."

We have to start protecting ourselves from the chemicals that come at us from every angle. This will not only help our hormone balance, it will also improve every aspect of our health. We can make a tremendous difference in our families' futures just by taking very small steps. Try a few of these, which were recommended by the Environmental Working Group (www.ewg.org).

- Avoid buying clothing advertised as stain-proof.
- Avoid microwaving food in plastic containers.
- Avoid drain cleaners; use a plumber's "snake" instead.
- Avoid nail care products containing dibutyl phthalate.
- Avoid products that include "fragrance" as an ingredient, because it commonly contains diethyl phthalate.

- Buy a polyethylene vinyl acetate (PEVA) biodegradable shower curtain or one made with cotton or another fabric.
- Look up where you can find the ingredient lists for your cleaning products at Ingredient Central, the Soap and Detergent Association's Web site (www.cleaning101.com/ingredientcentral).
- Don't choose products with stain-proof coatings, such as furniture and carpets.
- Don't let children put soft plastic toys in their mouths.
- Eat fewer greasy, prepackaged foods, which tend to be sold in containers coated with PFCs (perfluorinated chemicals).
- Get rid of Teflon and other nonstick pans.
- Use paints and other products that emit fumes in well-ventilated areas.
- Use vinegar, baking soda, and lemon—and a bit of elbow grease!—to clean your house.

This is merely the tip of the iceberg, but it's a start. Every little bit we can do to protect our bodies and our families from this toxic overload may be helpful. And as we start to demand products with fewer of these chemicals, these other industries—the cleaning product, cosmetics, even home design businesses—will be forced to comply. Or be left behind!

As we said at the beginning of this chapter, by far the biggest endocrine disruptor we're dealing with as a nation is excess weight. Many of the 5-minute fixes found throughout the book give you suggestions for how to manage your weight. But this is such an essential health aspect that we're devoting the entire next chapter to it. Let's get moving!

Chapter Eight

Take a Load Off

Earlier in the book, we talked about how life expectancy, for the first time in recorded history, is falling in the United States. One landmark study showed that many of the medical advances we've made in the past 100 years are being entirely offset by the damage done by obesity.

That study was done in 2005. But since then, it seems we haven't learned much, because the slide has continued unabated. In 2010, new research published in *The Lancet* looked at mortality rankings among 187 countries in the world and found that, while most countries' ranks have improved since 1990, in the United States, the risk of premature death continues to increase.

The United States is 45th in the world on the list of the countries with the lowest risk of death before age 60 among men; about 130 out of every 1,000 men in this country die before that age. When our women were compared with those in other countries, we ranked 49th, with 77 out of every 1,000 American women dying before their 60th birthdays.

Does that seem a little extreme to you? That 13 percent of the men in this country die before they're eligible for retirement?

We thought so, too.

Especially when we learned that that ranking put us behind less developed countries like Chile, Tunisia, and Albania. And way behind some European countries: Britain was 19th. Sweden was 2nd.

Now, how is it that in the country with the biggest gross domestic product, the country that spends by far the most money on health care, people have much shorter estimated life spans than people in Cuba? Or Libya?

What is going on here?

Perhaps most disturbing is how quickly our rankings have gotten worse. In 1990, our men were 41st; now they're 45th. Our women were 34th in the world; now they are *49th*. In 20 years, while global mortality has declined, the average US life span has plummeted.

And it's mostly attributable to excess weight.

Facing the Bull, Taking the Horns

How on earth could we have let this happen?

Throughout the book, we've talked about many factors that have led us to where we are. We talked about how we have many more calories readily available to us than ever before. We talked about insulin resistance and the toxic cycle of visceral fat. We've even talked about toxins in the environment and how many lead to hypothyroidism, diabetes, excess estrogen, and other conditions that can pack on weight.

At moments like this, we kind of wish we were magicians and could wave these things away. But we're not. We're medical doctors, and we have to deal in facts, logic, and science. And logic tells us that, regardless of the "obesogenic" (fat-promoting) environment that we find ourselves in, the only way we will collectively enjoy a healthy weight is if we acknowledge the jam we're in, agree that it stinks, and then agree to fight like hell not to let it claim us.

True, the government is working hard to regulate or ban some of the most dangerous risks, such as some of the chemicals, like bisphenol A, that are found in our food supply and some harmful foodstuffs, like hydrogenated fats. But we can't wait until we get the perfect environment with zero temptations, because we're never going to get that. No. What we have to do is face what we're given, take control, and take back our bodies.

And that starts right now.

Fix It in 5
Keep to a Healthy Weight

1. Cook your own whole foods rather than eating out.
2. Get help for any emotional eating.
3. Walk for 30 minutes, 5 days a week.
4. Eat a mix of carbs, protein, and fat at every meal and snack.
5. Watch the size of your portions.

A 5-Minute Tour of Healthy Weight Maintenance

Have you ever heard someone compare the human body to a bank? "When you eat, you make a deposit. When you exercise, you make a withdrawal," the analogy goes. "When you want to lose weight, just 'overdraw' your account—burn more calories than you consume—and you'll lose weight."

Sounds about right. We're lucky: We can turn food into fuel and store it for when we need it. It's a perfect strategy for when food supplies are limited, because it allows us to continue living our lives, using our reserves of fat for energy, without the need for a constant food supply. It works well—as long as our bodies are playing by the regular banking rules, that is.

But sometimes, things at the Healthy Weight Bank can get a bit off-kilter. Convenience stores and fast food restaurants are just down the street. Desk jobs keep us stationary for 9 or 10 hours a day.

Suddenly, our very innocent savings account can turn into a pyramid scheme: One extra snack turns into two. Two extra fat cells turn into four. Four extra pounds turn into 8, and so on and so on. Emboldened by a few extra pounds, your Bernie Madoff of a body can't stop—it gets addicted to "easy calories" and get-fat-quick schemes, and suddenly you're saddled with a whole lot more bad fat than you ever wanted.

What's a responsible health investor to do?

First of all, it's time to get back to basics and the body banking that suited us well for thousands of years. We're going to turn back the clock a bit, back before the time of low fat and low carb, before 30-second drive-thru guarantees and 3-minute microwave dinners. Instead of trying to save time with our meals, we're going to create some time—time to savor, enjoy, and nourish our bodies and our souls. It's time for some healthy weight sanity.

Keep It Simple

We love having Dr. Jim's dad, the legendary pediatrician and author William "Dr. Bill" Sears, MD, on the show. Recently he came on and shared with us his Rule of Twos:

Eat twice as often, eat half as much, and chew twice as long.

(Well, that about sums it up. Good night, everybody!)

Seriously—everything you need to know about how to stay at a healthy weight is in that sentence.

Eat twice as often. We are a nation that enjoys the idea of feast or famine. We skip meals and then we make up for it later. But this is a big mistake, especially when the meal we skip is breakfast. Eating breakfast is tremendously reliable indicator of a healthy weight. People who eat breakfast every day are *400 percent less likely to be obese* than those who skip it. Unfortunately, those who skip breakfast tend to "forget" to eat later as well—but then they make up for it by having a huge dinner at night. Right before bed. When they'll be flat on their backs for 8 hours.

What we need to do is follow Dr. Sears's advice and eat twice as often—three meals and two snacks a day, spaced 3 hours apart, will keep our metabolisms stoked and our blood sugars level. As we learned in Chapter 7, this balance is the key to preventing massive spikes of hunger and fat storage hormones.

Eat half as much. Our average daily consumption of calories has shot up by 523 calories over the last 40 years—from 2,234 to 2,757 since 1970. If we cut the sizes of our portions at any given meal in half, we would get back to portion sizes that are more like they were in 1970. In fact, if you are overweight and want to lose a few pounds and you could make only one change in the way you eat, this would be the one to make!

Chew twice as long. Dr. Sears means this both literally and figuratively. First, literally: When we chew food longer, each bite lasts longer, which prolongs the meal. The longer it takes us to eat our food, the less likely we are to overeat. By the time we're 30 minutes into the meal, a whole host of satiety hormones have had a chance to catch up with our chewing—hormones like peptide YY, which is produced by the digestive tract to signal the body that feeding time is over. When you chew for twice as long, as opposed to bolting down the first serving and getting seconds before this signal kicks in, you're likely to feel satisfied after eating less and be more apt to get up from the table.

Now, figuratively: Chewing twice as long can also be seen as a gentle reminder that we should slow down and enjoy our food. Enjoy the experience of eating, and the people you're eating with. Eating is not a task—it is one of life's great pleasures. We should not be concerned about saving time while eating; we should be doing what we can to create time. And there is no better way to create time than to be mindful of the moment and savor everything about it. Ultimately, we'll end up being way more satisfied after eating less food.

Keep It Real: The Good News

Here is perhaps the most surprising fact about achieving a healthy weight:

You may already be there.

Yes, obesity is the most common state of affairs. But recent research suggests that carrying around a bit of extra weight is not necessarily as devastating to your health as you may have been told. In fact, it might actually be healthier than any other body composition.

In a study published in *JAMA: The Journal of the American Medical Association*, researchers looked at the body mass indexes (BMIs) of hundreds of thousands of men and women and found, surprisingly, that those who fell into the overweight category—having a BMI of 25 to 29.9—actually had the lowest risk of mortality at any age, from 25 to more than 70. Even after 10 years of being overweight, their higher BMIs did not put them at any greater risk for mortality. In fact, these slightly overweight folks actually did a bit better than those who were in the normal range (from 18.5 to 24.9). The biggest risks of early mortality occurred in the underweight group (those whose BMIs were below 18.5) and the severely obese category (people with BMIs of more than 35).

So what does this mean for you? Well, if you're a 5-foot-6 woman who weighs 160 pounds (which gives you a BMI of 25.8) and you feel good, stop worrying. You don't have to kill yourself to lose those last 6 pounds to get down to 154 just to fit into the normal category. In fact, this research hints that it might not be that great of an idea.

Yes, people in the obese category should aim to lose some pounds. But could it be that "overweight" is the healthiest weight and "normal" is simply about aesthetics? We'll need more research to know for sure. But for now, it may be up to you to decide. We're not saying you should put on weight to get into the overweight category. We're just saying that as long as you feel comfortable in your skin and your BMI is not much higher than 26 or 27, you might just want to cut yourself a break.

The Bad News

Okay, so what if you aren't in that lucky zone of 26 or 27 BMI, but rather find yourself at 30, 31, or 32—what do you do? Take this opportunity to get a start on kicking that extra weight to the curb.

Obesity is bad news, friends. It may contribute to:

- back pain
- bladder problems
- bullying
- cancers: endometrial, breast, prostate, kidney, esophageal, uterine, and colon
- cognitive decline
- complications and infections after surgery
- depression
- discrimination
- eating disorders
- gallstones
- gout
- heart failure
- ineffective vaccination
- infertility in women
- kidney stones
- less success at work
- liver disease
- low self-esteem

I've been overweight my whole life. But even when I lose weight, it comes right back on. Why does it seem so hard for me to keep weight off? It just seems unfair.

You're right about the unfairness. You've undoubtedly noticed that some people seem to eat anything they want, whether they exercise or not, and never gain weight. Others, like you, tend to gain weight very easily and also struggle like you do to lose weight.

The weight controllers, like you, have many biological barriers to successful weight control. For example, when you lose weight, your fat cells (of which you have many billions more than your never-overweight peers), will shrink, but not disappear. They shrink and then they seem to impact certain cellular enzymes and hormones that promote weight gain. Those billions of extra fat cells act as if they were hungry baby sparrows with their mouths wide open—always looking for more food.

The good news is that *biology is not destiny*. You can learn to tame these biological barriers, but it won't be easy. Think about the challenges athletes face when learning how to run a 4-minute mile or hit tennis balls 120 mph with great accuracy. Their bodies resist those performances, just like your body resists weight loss. In both cases, disciplined training and focusing can overcome the biological barriers. Most people benefit from getting professional help, from experts trained in the physical and psychological challenges of weight loss, to develop the knowledge and skills necessary to succeed.

—**Dan Kirschenbaum, PhD, ABPP,** *director,*
Center for Behavioral Medicine & Sport Psychology, Northwestern University
Medical School, and author of The Healthy Obsession Program

- lower pay
- menstrual irregularity
- metabolic syndrome
- reduced brain volume
- type 2 diabetes

Obesity may cause up to 112,000 deaths a year in this country. If you gain 20 pounds between the ages of 18 and 40, you have double the risk of developing breast cancer after menopause. If you gain more than 22 pounds between the ages of 25 and 40, you increase your odds of having metabolic syndrome by 89 percent.

If you have never smoked cigarettes but you are obese at 50, your risk of death increases by 100 to 200 percent compared to your risk if your weight stays healthy.

Obesity: Definitely not a time-creator.

Okay, that's the situation—we know what we *don't* want. Now what are we going to do about it?

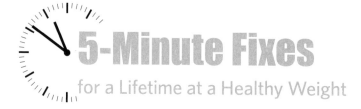

5-Minute Fixes
for a Lifetime at a Healthy Weight

Our objective for these 5-minute fixes is twofold:

1. If you are obese, we're going to work on taking off 10 percent of your weight. Once you're there, you'll take off another 10 percent, and then another 10, until you get into a healthy range for your body (see the BMI formula on page 288).

2. If you are at a healthy weight now, even if you are in that 25 to 27 BMI range and are happy with it, we'll help you hold the line against any future weight gain.

We're in luck—both of these objectives can be met with the lifestyle changes you'll find in these pages.

But before we begin, it is very important that you say it with us: "This is not a diet." While maintaining a healthy weight is important, everyone's healthy-weight threshold is different, and trying to force your body into meeting unrealistic weight goals can have devastating effects. A major complication of chronic dieting is weight cycling, where the dieter repeatedly loses and gains anywhere from 5 to 50 pounds. Research has linked this "yo-yo dieting" with high blood pressure, high cholesterol, and gallbladder disease.

With our 5-minute fixes, we're not asking you to "go on" a weight-loss program—that suggests you'll fall or go off it at some point. What we're hoping you'll do instead is make a series of permanent changes in the ways that you feed and move your body. And the best way to achieve that is with one small shift—one 5-minute fix—at a time.

By the Numbers: Obesity over the Ages

We're not imagining things when we look at kids today and think they're heavier than ever. A new study from the University of Michigan at Ann Arbor shows that what was previously thought of as age-related weight gain has instead been piling onto our youth.

OF PEOPLE BORN IN . . .	20 PERCENT WERE OBESE BY AGE . . .
1926–1935	50–59 years old
1936–1945	40–49 years old
1946–1955	30–39 years old
1966–1985	20–29 years old

Start with soda. This one's a no-brainer. If you cut out one absolutely nutritionally bankrupt can of soda per day, you could lose almost 15 pounds in 1 year. Fifteen pounds! If you're a soda addict and you can't imagine going without, consider that in the years between 1970 and 1990, our consumption of soda went up by 86 percent and our obesity rate rose by 112 percent. Coincidence? Doubtful. Researchers have found that when you drink soda, you lose the ability to regulate your own calories for the rest of the day. Sodas and other foods containing high-fructose corn syrup may not register in your satiety center, or they may make you hungrier, or they just may make you crave more and more sweets. The Framingham Heart Study found that drinking more than one 12-ounce soda a day can significantly increase the risk of developing high blood pressure. Other

I've tried everything to lose weight,
but I have not been successful. How do I know
if I'm a good candidate for stomach stapling?

Bariatric surgery—such as gastric bypass (sometimes formerly referred to as stomach stapling), gastric banding, and other procedures that reroute your digestive tract to make your stomach smaller and reduce your absorption of calories—is an option for people who are severely obese and have been unable to lose weight by dieting and exercising, or who have serious weight-related health problems. Here's what to consider.

Your weight: According to the National Institutes of Health (NIH), you may be a candidate if you're a man who is 100 pounds overweight or a woman who is 80 pounds overweight. This means having a body mass index (BMI)—a measurement that relates your height and weight—of 40 or more. (Find out what your BMI is by using the NIH's online calculator at www.nhlbisupport.com/bmi or the formula on page 288.)

Weight-related medical conditions: Weight-loss surgery may be right for you if you have a BMI

research has linked drinking soda to high triglycerides and lower HDL levels. Any way you look at it, it's poison. **Time spent:** 5 minutes emptying all of the soda bottles and cans in the house into the sink and putting them in the recycling bin—they will be gone before you know it

If you must have a soda, double (or triple!) the glass size. Okay, we know that some people can't live without their daily 16 ounces of soda. While we'd love for you to just go cold turkey, here's one way you can lessen the impact of the sugar while also getting some extra hydration. Take a 32-ounce glass, pack it with ice, and then pour the can or bottle into that glass. You'll still get the treat, but it will last longer and, by the time the ice melts and you've finished the glass, you'll have an extra 16 or 20 ounces of water in your body as well. **Time spent:** 10 seconds to grab a glass and pack in some ice, 30 seconds to pour

of 35 or higher and have a serious obesity-related medical condition such as arthritis, type 2 diabetes, high blood pressure, high cholesterol, sleep apnea, or a family history of early heart disease. (For people with type 2 diabetes, some researchers say that having a BMI of 30 to 32 makes you a good candidate for surgery.)

Your age: Surgery is generally recommended for people between the ages of 20 and 60. But teens and older people may also benefit. (Be sure that you and your doctor talk through all the risks of the surgery, both in regard to your age as well as other risk factors.)

Your readiness for change: Bariatric surgery is a weight-loss tool—you'll shed pounds only if you stick with the low-calorie diet and regular exercise program recommended by your doctor after your procedure. The University of California at San Francisco reports that gastric bypass patients lose an average of 77 percent of their excess weight in the year after surgery. Other studies have found some patients keep 50 to 60 percent of their extra weight off for 10 to 14 years.

Your general health: Surgery always has risks. Experts say that people with severe heart or kidney disease aren't good candidates. Infections, health conditions that could cause bleeding in your stomach or esophagus, diseases of your liver or pancreas, and having a risk of alcoholism and drug addiction also indicate that surgery may not be right for you.

*—**Ritu Chopra, MD,** Beverly Hills plastic surgeon, and **Dr. Drew Ordon***

Stop counting calories (if you're a woman over 65). Finally, right? Here's the thing: It may be better for you to stay at your current weight than to lose more, especially when it comes to your bones. Older women who lose weight can double their risk of hip fracture. If you're dead set on losing weight, just be sure to get adequate calcium by drinking three or four glasses of fat-free or low-fat milk per day (or the equivalent), and definitely get your exercise in. You might want to choose weight-bearing exercise, like walking with hand weights, over the gentler but not bone-preserving aqua aerobics. **Time spent:** 30 minutes a day of walking (although you'll save 20 minutes during the rest of your day if you stop counting calories)

Stand up for yourself. Consider asking your workplace's facilities or maintenance group if the height of your desk can be raised so you can stand in front of it to work. According to the *American*

Journal of Preventive Medicine, people who spend more than 6 hours a day in a chair are 68 percent more likely to become overweight. But a recent study from the University of Missouri–Columbia found that standing up and walking around can stimulate lipoprotein lipase, an enzyme, to scour your blood for fat (to turn it into energy) and cholesterol (to change it from LDL into heart-healthy HDL). If you're just sitting around, slouching into your computer, this activity could plummet by 90 percent and your blood would soon be swimming in fat—no higher HDL for you.

If you're not able to adapt your desk, maybe just make it a habit to stand while you're on the phone or reading an article. Or you could go to the supply room and lift (some reams of paper, that is), bring the mail up from the mailroom, or take the recycling outside. These tasks may not be part of your job description, but they take a bit of energy (aka calories burned), and, bonus, they'll win you pals and get you out of the office, into the vitamin D–producing sun! **Time spent:** shoot for at least an hour a day to start, just 5 minutes at a time!

Chew each bite 20 times. One study of more than 3,000 Japanese adults published in the *British Medical Journal* found that those who ate quickly were roughly twice as likely to become obese—regardless of how many calories they ate. The same study looked at the effect of "eating until full" and found it had the same effect—and when combined, these two bad habits increased the subjects' chances of being overweight by about 220 percent. Take your time—you'll eat less and most likely feel feel vastly more satisfied. **Time spent:** 20 seconds for each bite

Drink a glass of Oregon pinot noir. A large-scale study of nearly 20,000 women ages 39 and over found that those who drank 1 ounce of alcohol a day—one serving of beer, wine, or hard alcohol—were the least likely to become overweight or obese. In fact, they had a 30 percent lower risk than those who abstained. Curiously enough, the women who did not drink alcohol gained the most weight, but as soon as a woman started drinking again, she lost weight. The strongest connection was with red wine.

I want our kids to be fit and healthy, so they can avoid childhood obesity. Any tips?

Dr. Jim says . . .

You bet! I've got millions. I'm so worried because the prevalence of obesity in children jumped up 10 percent in just 4 years. In just girls, it was an 18 percent rise! We are at a crisis point. But these tips will work for the whole family—Mom and Dad, too.

1. No soda. Period. The end. No more discussion.

2. Water down juices and fruit punches. Or have them full-strength only on very "special" occasions, such as birthday parties. The average American over 2 years old consumes 132 calories every day from high-fructose corn syrup, which is almost criminal, but even 100 percent juice is incredibly high in natural sugars.

3. Allow free eating of "grow food." Stock your kitchen with yogurt, carrots, cheese sticks, apples, bananas, popcorn. Once kids get to an age where they can feed themselves, allow them ready access to those foods, on their schedule. You want them to listen to their own hunger cues. As long as they're getting a good variety of healthy foods, try not to get frustrated if they just nibble at dinner. The sooner they "own" their hunger, the less likely they'll be to give in to junk food bingeing later on.

4. Encourage outdoor play. Get a trampoline, a jungle gym. Buy roller skates, balls, Frisbees. Take them to parks. And let them explore, even if it makes you nervous. Your children have an infinitesimal chance of being gravely hurt or abducted—but if you don't allow them out of the house, they have a much greater chance of becoming obese, which will put them at higher risk for being bullied and developing depression.

5. Walk them to school. The American Academy of Pediatrics recommends 1 hour of vigorous activity for kids every day—but very few get that. Set up a "walking bus" and collect kids from the neighborhood. If you drive your kids to school, park a half-mile away and walk them the rest of the way. Build this natural exercise into their day and they'll burn off energy (and calories) before school, be more focused and ready to work, and develop a lifelong exercise habit, to boot. Oregon instituted a "walk to school" program that, along with other initiatives, lowered that state's childhood obesity rate by 32 percent.

Go for a pinot noir from the Oregon coast—that particular grape grown in that particular region has been shown to have one of the highest levels of resveratrol of any wine. Resveratrol is an antioxidant that helps reduce LDL cholesterol and prevent blood clots and damage to the blood vessels. It may also help manage diabetes and reduce beta-amyloid plaque in our brains, a biomarker for Alzheimer's. Now that's what we call a powerhouse fix! **Time spent:** as many delightful minutes as you'd like per glass

Put a bowl of sugar-free gum on the counter. Sometimes, what's right in front of you can save the day. If you have kids, or just a vicious sweet tooth, having a bowl of sugar-free gum ready and waiting can head off a lot of "Can I have a treat?" whining (from both of you). Sugar-free gum with xylitol can help manage plaque, making it a great way to finish off a meal instead of reaching for dessert. And one study actually found that you can burn calories by chewing gum. Not many, mind you—only 11 per hour—but still!

If this tip is really working for you—and you're a gum-chewing fiend—look for a brand without sorbitol. Too much could give you a case of the runs. **Time spent:** 5 seconds to unwrap a piece and enjoy

Reward your first few pounds lost with some new sheets. After how and how much you exercise your body and how many calories you put into it, the third most important variable in controlling your weight is how much you sleep. When we don't get enough sleep, we interrupt many important metabolic-hormone processes. After just 1 night of sleep deprivation, our levels of leptin—a hormone that helps control appetite and boosts metabolism—start to take a hit. When sleep is restricted for 2 nights, the hunger hormone ghrelin increases by 28 percent. Sleep apnea and other disturbances can put us at higher risk for insulin resistance and higher levels of neuropeptide Y, an appetite-increasing chemical in our brains.

Sleep shouldn't be a luxury we allow ourselves when we have enough time. Take a hint from Hollywood celebs who make plenty of shut-eye the very first item in their beauty regimen. You just might be saving your own life—a recent study found that those of us who get less than 6 hours of sleep a night have a much greater chance of early death. Hit the sheets!

Time spent: 5 minutes to pick out a nice pair of 300-thread-count (or higher) sheets online, then 7 to 8 hours a night, no excuses

Turn down your air conditioner. We know this one won't be popular. But consider it your gift to the earth and your waistline at the same time. Heat is nature's appetite suppressant. There's a reason that we tend to eat light foods in the summer—it feels yucky to process heavy creams and gravies when it's 90°F outside. When hotter air temperatures raise your core body temperature, it increases your metabolic rate by 7 to 17 percent. But our culture's addiction to air-conditioning robs us of this effect on two levels: by making it unseasonably cool—and therefore fine weather for overeating—as well as by preventing our bodies from ever feeling that heat. **Time spent:** 10 minutes to adjust your air conditioner's automatic timer to give yourself an hour or two to really feel the heat (and the burn!) every summer day

Finish a workout, eat a chicken breast. A study done at the University of Michigan found that each session of aerobic exercise enhances your insulin sensitivity—especially when the meal you eat right after it is low in carbs. Researchers found that the effect doesn't last very long—just a few hours or, at most, a few days. But the beauty is, you can reap the same insulin-related benefits as someone who chooses a lower-calorie but higher-carb postworkout snack. Eat more and get the same health benefits? Sign us up! Skip the banana and stick to a handful of nuts, a cup of cottage cheese, or a protein bar. **Time spent:** 3 minutes packing a high-protein snack before you head to the gym; 5 minutes to nibble on it after you hit the mat

Shoot for 12 miles. This is the distance that researchers at Duke University in Durham, North Carolina, discovered you should walk every week if you want to prevent any more accumulation of visceral fat, the toxic belly fat that leads to increased inflammation and heart disease risks. Sound like a lot? That depends on your current level of fitness, but the researchers tested the program on a group of sedentary folks who either walked or ran 12 miles a week. Both groups held the line against new fat—and the members of a third group that ran 20 miles a week were able to decrease it.

Start with about 2 miles a day, 5 days a week, for a few weeks. If you're feeling spry, and have your doctor's okay, start a run/walk program: Run for 1 minute, then walk for 1 minute, and keep alternating for the full 2 miles. Continue to increase the running time and decrease the walking time—or bump up your workout time by 5 minutes here and there—and you'll sail past that 12-mile mark in no time. **Time spent:** 20 minutes a day if you're jogging or 30 to 40 minutes a day if you're walking, 5 days a week

Ban the butt. If you have a pal (or a spouse!) who's been stinking up the joint with his or her smokes, consider this your reason to boot them to the porch: Secondhand smoke raises your risk of glucose intolerance (a risk factor for diabetes) by 35 percent—almost the same as smoking itself. We're sure that if you explain it, your pal will understand that you don't want to "catch" diabetes from his or her smokes. And who knows? You might even inspire the person to quit! **Time spent:** 5 minutes for a good laying-down-the-law chat

Hire a buddy. Sometimes all we need to make a positive change is a kick in the pants—or 12. A study from the University of Michigan published in the journal *Preventive Medicine* looked

DOCTOR, DOCTOR, GIMME THE NEWS: DIHYDROCAPSIATE—FEEL THE BURN WITHOUT THE BURNING FEELING

You may have heard that capsaicin, the source of the heat in chile peppers, can temporarily turn up the heat on your metabolism. That's all well and good for those of us who like spicy food—but what about those whose palates go for milder tones? Good news: Researchers at the UCLA Center for Human Nutrition who tested a nonburning version of capsaicin, dihydrocapsiate, found that, at high doses, it significantly increased calorie burning (by twice as much as a placebo did), as well as increasing the body's fat-burning activity. Like a case of post-Mexican-food heartburn, the effect is short-lived—but we'll take it! While not on the market just yet, a dihydrocapsiate product is pending FDA approval—and we'll be sure to cover it on the show as soon as it hits.

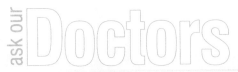

ask our **Doctors**

Why do I find it so hard to stop eating junk food? Could I be "addicted" to sugar?

The evidence is pretty strong that we can, in fact, be addicted—or nearly so—to sugar, as well as salt, and dietary fat. Cravings for such nutrients actually make sense, but only in context.

Throughout most of human history, getting any of these nutrients was challenging, and beneficial. Salt is an essential nutrient, sugar provides quick energy, and fat is the most concentrated source of calories. Junk foods provide in abundance the very items our Stone Age survival taught us to favor. With any addictive-like tendency, the more you get, the more you need. So if you bathe your taste buds in sugar, salt, and fats all day, you will need more and more to get satisfaction.

The good news here is that this works in reverse, as well; purify your diet incrementally, and you can rehabilitate your taste buds. Start by taking sugar out of your diet where it least belongs—pasta sauces, salad dressings, crackers, bread—and as you need less and less of the sweet stuff for satisfaction, you will be able to dial down the sweet junk foods as well.

—**David Katz, MD, MPH, FACPM, FACP,** *director, Prevention Research Center at the Yale University School of Medicine and author of* Dr. David Katz's Flavor-Full Diet

at what would happen if people who were trying to increase their intake of vegetables received three counseling calls from a dietitian compared to others who were given nutritional literature, but didn't receive those calls. After 12 weeks, the folks who had had the friendly chats had made significantly greater changes to their diets, adding more fruits and vegetables. They also increased their blood levels of carotenoids—which are antioxidants—by 20 percent. The people who received only educational materials with or without a diet plan did not show the same improvements.

This study proves something we all know intuitively: When we're trying to make changes

Take a Load Off   **195**

in our lives, support really helps. We know that not everyone has the means to hire a personal trainer or nutritionist—in fact, most of us don't. Instead, consider going online to a virtual assistant Web site like Elance.com and hiring a professional nagger, someone who will call you every few weeks to check on your progress. More reliable than a friend and cheaper than a trainer, you'll at least know someone is watching out for you! **Time spent:** 5 minutes online to post your job, 5 minutes to collect and review the bids, and 5 minutes per phone call to stay on track!

ask our Doctors

I've heard so much about the different diets out there—low fat, low carb, vegan, etc. Is there one program that's better than another?

A couple of clinical trials have shown that, over a two-year period, it doesn't matter which diet you use, low-carb or high-carb—what's more important is that you show up for weight loss group meetings and you reduce calories. The actual composition of the diet doesn't matter. People can feel free to make personal choices.

Of course, I'm not saying to consume a low-calorie diet of soda! But *which* healthy diet doesn't make any difference. Bottom line, reduce your intake of energy-dense foods with added sugar or added fat, fried foods, and reduce portion size. Choose high-fiber fruits and veggies and low-fat dairy.

No matter what your culture or food preference is, it's important that you recognize that food is tied to your family and lifestyle. Too often there is a message that "diet" food has to look like it came from another planet and that puts people off. But lowering calories and increasing activity can work within the context of any culture or diet.

—*Elizabeth Mayer-Davis, MSPH, PhD, RD,* president-elect,
health care and education, American Diabetes Association

Avoid the fast food mile. Every town has a street clogged with these hangouts. But you may not realize that just driving down that street and seeing the signs and logos—even if you don't stop—could be sabotaging your long-term health—and even financial!—goals.

Three separate experiments that researchers at the University of Toronto did with 57 college students showed a link between exposure to fast food logos and impatience. During one of the experiments, the students were shown either pictures of the fast food logos or signs from other, nonchain restaurants. The students "primed" with the corporate logos had a much lower level of interest in saving money. When combined with the results of the other two experiments, the researchers concluded that priming people with these logos led them to seek more immediate gratification ("I want my Cinnabon, and I want it *now*!"). They also read faster and had more interest in saving time.

Remember what we said about slowing down. Fast food is the ultimate in mindless eating. Avoid any exposure to that toxic mind-set—and metabolic nightmare. **Time spent:** 5 minutes avoiding the fast food mile; it could be worth it in the long run

Steer clear of the newspaper recipe section. A small study looked at the recipe sections of all the newspapers published in three cities that had 400,000 or more residents. Researchers picked the last week of August in 2000 and looked at the recipes for entrees, desserts, snacks, and appetizers and analyzed their nutritional content. They found that the desserts' calorie counts reflected perfectly the reported obesity rates for the area. When the recipes were fatty and calorie-laden, the local community tended to have higher rates of obesity. When the content was leaner and healthier, the rates of obesity were lower.

While this study doesn't show whether the recipes started the trends or the newspapers' editors were astute observers of their towns' tastes instead, it's certainly a good wake-up call that we need to look for the healthiest recipes we can find for lean dishes and salads. Be a good neighbor and bring a healthy dish to the next potluck—or submit a healthy recipe to the paper for publication. Who knows, you might start a health trend in your town. **Time spent:** 5 minutes to peruse the recipe section and think, "Hmm, are we a fit or fat town?"

Drs' Orders
for a Healthy Weight:
Eat Smaller Portions

We know, we know—we all hate to cut calories. And who can blame us? Who wants to spend life with a fork in one hand and a calculator in the other?

That's why Dr. Sears's suggestion to eat half as much is such a good one. You don't have to look at food labels or review the nutrition facts. You simply eyeball your serving, cut it in half, and away you go. Of course, we're presuming that you're making wise nutritional decisions in the first place—half of a fried chicken is not exactly what we have in mind here. But if you focus on cutting refined carbs and high-fat meats in half and filling in the space with an array of colorful vegetables (mostly green), you'll have gone a long way toward automatic weight loss.

None of us should think of this as deprivation; instead, we should think of it as dialing back on one of the modern advances that has not served us well: overserving. We all tend to reach for a certain amount out of habit when the serving dish is placed in front of us. If we could simply stop that act of automatic serving, step back to take a good look at it, and cut it in half, we'd be doing ourselves a tremendous favor. Other ways we can reduce portion sizes automatically, without feeling deprived:

- Use smaller plates, bowls, and cups.
- Order half portions or appetizer portions of entrees in restaurants (or ask the waitress to wrap half to go).
- Double the vegetables and halve the starch.
- Order the kid's meal—with extra vegetables.
- Try starting every dinner with a non-creamy soup or vinaigrette-dressed salad, no exceptions.

- Buy 100-calorie packs for small treats.
- Stay away from soda!

The bottom line is that, as a culture, we have to get away from thinking about food as a means of comfort or using it to fill an emotional void. It is a pleasure, but it is one of many in a healthy, well-rounded life. Friends, family, loved ones . . . all are more important than shoveling more junk down our throats. We need to work on how we can find a sense of peace in our connection with these people, as well as foster contentment within ourselves in other ways that don't involve food. Let's take a look, though, at what is perhaps the most important determinant of our health: our relationships.

Chapter Nine
Love Will Keep Us Together

We've talked about the huge effect stress can have on you physically and the benefits of stress relief. But more and more scientific evidence is piling up that good relationships, in and of themselves, benefit your health—possibly more than almost any other health behavior.

Of course, the most important relationship you have is the one you have with yourself: If you don't value your self and your body, you're less likely to take care of your health and more likely to fall into destructive habits that will cut your life short, like smoking, drinking, or abusing drugs—or even overeating and underexercising.

Volumes have been written about the human condition, and we could fill a library with tomes describing the different philosophies about how our emotions and our relationships impact our health. We're going to focus on a few emotions that can be major influences on your health—both for the good and for the bad—and how those emotions can help shape not only your sense of self-worth and your relationships, but also the trajectory of your entire life.

Fix It in 5
Create a Health-Giving Positive Attitude

1. Be grateful.
2. Savor the moment.
3. Use your strengths and do what you love.
4. Love yourself as you are—and connect with others who do the same.
5. Take a deep breath and count to 10 before you react.

A 5-Minute Tour of Your Emotional Health

You have probably heard that certain emotions, like hostility and explosive anger, are not good for your health. Studies have linked hostile emotions to increased risks of high blood pressure and heart disease, greater amounts of visceral fat and systemic inflammation, and an overall risk of earlier death. One study found that a higher level of what the authors called "destructive anger" was associated with a 31 percent greater risk of coronary heart disease in both men and women. Makes sense, right? These are the road-rage poster children. You can practically see their veins popping out of their foreheads.

But it might surprise you to know that sometimes a quieter emotion, one that's at the opposite end of the "acting out" spectrum, can be equally if not more dangerous: hopelessness. If you have ever felt that there is no point to your life, that you do not have control over your destiny, and that your efforts will not result in the outcomes you hope for, then you have met hopelessness. Let's make sure it doesn't become a close friend and you'll be just fine.

Researchers have begun to discover that when people feel hopeless, their ability to fight off illness, indeed their entire physical well-being, can be put in jeopardy. And when you mix anger and hopelessness together—you are angry at the world because you believe "there's no point, no one cares anyway"—you have a particularly toxic cocktail, one that increases your blood pressure and dramatically threatens your health.

The Power of the Word

Now, we ask you: When you read that phrase—"there's no point, no one cares anyway"—did it make your heart sink a little? Did it make you feel a little depressed, a little weaker?

No wonder. Scientists are learning more every day about how language creates our thoughts.

A recent study from Germany proved that hearing the words "This is going to hurt" before we get a shot triggers the pain response in our brains—we actually feel pain before the needle even touches the skin! Researchers used functional MRI to study people's brains and found that their pain centers lit up like pinball machines when they heard words that suggested intense pain was coming.

What this tells us is that words matter. When we say or listen to words conveying negative or painful thoughts or feelings, our brains immediately activate to feel that pain. In some ways, this is an amazingly human trait—we are very empathetic creatures. But there are situations where that compassion—even for ourselves—might cause problems. When a person with chronic pain talks about her pain with a support group, the close relationships and understanding she finds there are certain to help her. But if during those meetings, she "shares" how she's been struggling, might she actually be reinforcing that pain in herself and others? It's certainly a valid question.

Whatever the answer, this area of research demonstrates one thing clearly: We have a tremendous ability to control our own health destinies simply by changing our internal dialogue. Consider this chain of events: Think positive thoughts. Say positive words. Surround yourself with positive people. What will happen? Your body will eagerly drink in all the corresponding health benefits: lower blood pressure, lower levels of stress hormones, increased amounts of health-promoting neurotransmitters and hormones like dopamine, endorphins, and oxytocin.

Now, that doesn't mean we're all going to have to turn into Stuart Smalley, Al Franken's *Saturday Night Live* character whose trademark line—"I'm good enough, I'm smart enough, and doggone it, people like me"—gave personal mantras a bit of a bad rep. But I think we can agree that the research is clear: Stuart in his own bumbling way was on to something.

If we can learn to take those two negative emotions—hostility and hopelessness—and consciously turn them into their positive cousins—gratitude and resilience—we'll have taken the first step. Our internal words create our thoughts, those thoughts create our feelings, those feelings create physical effects. We have a choice about whether those physical effects will be positive or negative. We have a choice about what we say to ourselves—and we can make this entire mind–body chain reaction work for us instead of against us. (Admit it: The thought "I am so grateful for my husband!" is much more pleasant to feel than "He's so selfish. Nobody cares about me," isn't it?)

If we practice every day, we can retrain our brains to seek out the good and appreciate it (gratitude), while we learn from our experiences and continue to grow in a positive direction (resilience). Because our minds absorb and reflect the emotions of those who surround us, we will suddenly find that we're way more fun to be around.

WHAT YOUR BODY'S TRYING TO TELL YOU: SOCIAL ANXIETY

Feel scared before walking into a party or talking to a large group of people? You're not alone. Some 15 million Americans have social anxiety that makes them feel extremely self-conscious in the company of friends and strangers at work, at school, and in other purely social situations.

Almost everybody gets a few butterflies before meeting new people or standing up to make a speech. But if social anxiety interferes with your life—or if you find you're relying on alcohol or drugs to cope—counseling can help. Studies show that a short-term, solution-focused approach called cognitive-behavioral therapy helps three out of four people reduce their social anxiety.

Signs and symptoms include:

- A persistent, intense, and chronic fear of being judged and evaluated by other people
- Blushing
- Sweating
- Trembling
- Nausea
- Difficulty talking in social situations

Cognitive-behavioral therapy is a systematic approach that helps you reframe your negative thoughts into positive ones. Some people see improvements after just a few sessions. It's like having a personal trainer for your brain—try it!

Healthy people like being around healthy people.

What comes next might even be the most powerful and longest-lasting benefit. We'll be much better spouses, friends, lovers, and co-workers, which will enhance our relationships so we can benefit from what healthy-aging studies have identified as the single most important positive health factor: warm, supportive connections to people we love. It's been found that divorced or widowed people and those in bad relationships have 20 percent more chronic health conditions, and people in good marriages and strong families tend to live 4 to 6 years longer than people who don't.

Now, truth be told, for those relationships to last and flourish, they'll need a bit more of our elbow grease and sustained attention than just a liberal application of good attitude can provide. So we'll include two go-to techniques that you can employ in any relationship, whether it's with your spouse or your hairdresser, to help everyone win: Practice acceptance. And set healthy boundaries.

When we truly accept people and show them that our love for them won't change regardless of their behavior or opinions, it reaffirms their basic worth and they feel more loved. They see that we're not trying to change them or make them into anything they're not; they simply *are*, and that's good enough for us.

Acceptance is tough, and certainly not the end of the story. We can't accept all behavior, especially when it's unhealthy for us (or for our kids, if we're tasked with taking care of a little person). We also need some protection for when others are not accepting of *us*—we can't just accept other people's judgments of us if they don't fit. So that's why we need to have the skill to set boundaries. Healthy boundaries allow us to be fun and spontaneous and open and loving, but also responsible for our own needs. We need to know what our own limits are so we can communicate them clearly to others.

All of these changes sound good, right? But they are easy to say and a bit tougher to put into practice. And we do say "practice" because, just like any of the other fixes in this book, changing your mind-set and your relationships isn't about waking up one morning and saying, "Right! On with this new way!"

Instead, we need to make these changes in one 5-minute chunk at a time. We need to face hundreds and eventually thousands of challenging personal and social situations and, each time, simply say, "I don't have to be angry. I can be calm. I can be grateful."

And, "I don't have to let this flatten me," and then pick yourself up, point yourself in a different direction, and start again.

And, "I don't agree with his opinion, but it's his and he is entitled to it. It doesn't make me love him less!"

And, "I don't really feel comfortable with that. But thanks for asking."

Trust us: Seemingly small decisions like this, made dozens of times each day, will eventually bring about tremendous changes—in yourself and in your relationships with everyone in your world.

Okay. We've got work to do! Our 5-minute fixes in this chapter will focus on all of these means of positive reframing: Taking what was negative and turning it into a positive. In so doing, we have the power to reshape our families, our relationships with our loved ones, and our health.

5-Minute Fixes
for a Lifetime of Positive Relationships

Studies from every culture on earth prove it: Good relationships with friends, colleagues, and family keep you healthy (and of course happy!) in a variety of ways.

No matter if you're young or old, single or married, the life of the party or a total hermit, if you focus on fostering gratitude and resilience, if you accept yourself and other people the way they are, and if you set healthy boundaries, you can use these traits to connect with others and build better relationships, creating a chain of health that you and all those you meet can link to for a lifetime.

Fix that communication breakdown. Good communication is one of the hallmarks of—and most important skills in—close relationships. And honest, respectful communication is such a time-saver! When you say what you mean the first time, you avoid misunderstandings, fights, and hurt feelings that can drag on for days, months, or years.

KNOW WHERE YOU STAND

	PASSIVE	ASSERTIVE	AGGRESSIVE
Behavior	Ignores and does not express rights, needs, and desires	Makes "I" statements	Makes "you" statements
	Permits others to infringe upon his or her rights	Expresses and asserts own rights, needs, and desires	Expresses him- or herself at the expense of others
	Is emotionally dishonest, indirect, inhibited	Stands up for legitimate rights in a way that does not violate the rights of others	Has inappropriate outbursts or hostile overreactions, humiliates or "gets even" with others, puts others down
	Is self-denying	Is emotionally honest, direct, expressive	Emotionally honest, direct, expressive—at others' expense
	Is self-demeaning	Is self-enhancing	Is self-enhancing
	Allows others to choose	Chooses for self	Chooses for others
Feelings That Result	Hurt, anxiety, disappointment in self at the time and possibly angry later	Confidence, self-respect, satisfaction with self at the time and later	Angry, then self-righteous, superior, derogatory, possibly guilty later
Outcomes	Does not achieve desired goal(s)	May achieve desired goal(s)	Achieves desired goal(s) by hurting others
Payoffs	Avoids risky situations; avoids conflict, tension, confrontation; doesn't have needs met; accumulates anger; feels unvalued	Feels good, feels valued by self and others, feels better about self, has improved self-confidence, has needs met, has relationships that are freer and more honest	Saves up anger, feels that resentment justifies a blowup or emotional outburst, gets even with or gets back at people

Source: Judith A. Belmont, *The Therapeutic Companion* (Allentown, PA: Worksite Insights, 2007)

My mom gave me some serious body-image
issues that I've struggled with my entire life.
I am terrified that I'm going to repeat the same
patterns with my daughter. What can I do to
make sure she grows up to be confident in herself?

Dr. Lisa says . . .

First, let me just say what a great mom you are! The fact that you're even asking this question shows that your daughter will have an easier time of it than you did.

What's tricky is that you have to balance teaching her about responsible eating and exercise with not making her self-conscious about her body. You need to accept her for who she is and honor her personal boundaries so she can develop them on her own. All parents struggle with this, and the matter is typically complicated by our own histories, attitudes, and body-image issues. Here's what I suggest.

Supply the food and walk away. It's the parent's job to bring healthy food into the house; it's the kid's job to put it into her body. Do not urge, bribe, command, or otherwise coerce your child to eat. If this attempt to control her food intake becomes a battle of wills, she will either rebel, refusing to eat and then sneaking snacks, or she'll comply and eat when she's not hungry.

Human communication exists on a continuum. At one end is the person who is passive, who doesn't respect himself enough to ask for what he needs. At the other end is someone who is aggressive, who takes what she needs without any respect for the other person. The middle way, assertiveness, is the land of healthy communication. And that's where we want to live.

Many of us think we're assertive, that we try to get our needs met without bullying or going belly up. The chart on page 209 will help you figure out where you stand on the passive–assertive–aggressive spectrum. You may be surprised by what category you find some of your most favored thought patterns and attitudes in. Chances are, you'll find you fall into each of the columns, sometimes during the same conversation.

Either way, she'll learn to turn off her hunger cues in response to external signals.

Don't force her to hug or kiss anyone. If she won't give grandma a hug, don't insist. If you teach her from a very early age to be in charge of her body, she won't have to "relearn" it as a teen or adult.

Don't call attention to her body. "You're so slim—look at those long legs! Boy, I wish I had a body like yours. I'd have to diet for a year to look like that." Ban this kind of talk. Even complimentary messages give girls the feeling that they're being judged on their looks. And though they are by others, they don't have to be by you! There's plenty of time for that in our culture; protect her from judgments, even those coming from well-meaning relatives. Pull your mother-in-law aside and explain the rules to her. If she thinks you're ridiculous—"I was being nice!"—thank her, but reiterate your stand.

Avoid putting yourself down. "I can't believe I have to put a bathing suit on in 3 weeks! Ugh. Hideous." No. She is listening; everything that comes out of your mouth goes straight into her brain. You may have to work on your automatic scripts about your body, but you must refrain from these monologues.

Let her pick out her own clothes from a young age. From the moment she can select her own socks, allow her to put together the craziest ensembles she can find. This daily process of figuring out how she wants to present herself to the world is excellent practice. She'll learn that she owns her body, that it's her responsibility, and that what she wants to show people is all that matters. When the stripes and the polka dots toddle down the stairs, bite your tongue—and see the proud young woman who's soon to be!

You might want to memorize a few of these telltale signs to help you manage conflict. Becoming aware of how you communicate is the first step in reaching healthy assertiveness because it makes it easier to resist the urge to swing to either of the poles. Steer yourself toward the center of the chart, and your relationships will surely benefit. **Time spent:** 30 seconds to check in with yourself and make a mental note about your language each time you are in an uncomfortable conversation

Urge your teen to take a nap. In a study funded by the National Institutes of Health, researchers from the University of California at San Diego looked at the social networks of

I've been in a funk for a while now. Even my husband is starting to say, "You should go see someone." But how do I know if it's time to see a therapist or if I can just shake it off?

Dr. Jim says . . .

When you feel mentally under the weather, it's really hard to get perspective. Are you just having a few "down days" or are you depressed? You might want to feel better and may even be asking yourself, "What's my problem—why can't I just get it together?" It's not unusual to have periods of explained or unexplained sadness for a few days or even for a week. But if you feel like you're slugging through day after day for an extended period of time, such as two weeks or more, you could be depressed. If you feel indifferent or your mental and physical energy has dropped down and it's making it hard to get your work done or spend time with your family, then you might need to seek help. Is your mood impacting you in a negative way, affecting your relationships, or keeping your from accomplishing things you want to accomplish? Your are your own best barometer. Keep your eye out for warning signs, which might include the following:

- Can't sleep or sleeping all the time
- Disruption in normal eating pattern (overeating or not eating at all)

8,349 adolescents in grades 7 through 12. They found that groups of kids who had bad sleep habits also tended to use marijuana—and that both of those habits had actually spread to other kids within their networks. While, traditionally, parents and school officials would focus on eradicating the drug use first, these researchers found that when parents encouraged better sleep habits—by taking the TV out of the child's bedroom, limiting computer and phone usage to daytime and early evening hours, and encouraging napping—those changes actually had a greater impact on the girls' drug use—and, by extension, on their friends'.

- Crying spells or not being able to cry
- Loss of interest or pleasure in people or activities that you used to enjoy
- Feeling alone, even when people are around
- Having no energy or motivation to do things that might make you feel better
- Lack of focus and/or concentration
- Feeling worthless
- Hopelessness
- Feeling that the world would be better off without you
- Slowed speech
- Thoughts of death or suicide
- Feeling fatigued
- Guilt that prevents you from enjoying anything
- Feeling sad and empty about what you haven't accomplished in life or what you may accomplish in the future.

If you have any of these symptoms, it could be depression—and you might think about seeing someone. A therapist or psychologist could help figure out if a specific problem is bugging you, or if you have a wider problem. Even one session can help sometimes.

If you feel more comfortable talking to your regular doctor, that can be a good first step as well. Just let them know that you've not been feeling like yourself lately. They can help get you started, to determine if you should go see a therapist or a psychiatrist. There are several effective ways to relieve your symptoms. You don't have to struggle anymore. Reach out and talk—and you may find the solution is very close at hand.

If your kid is using drugs, this might be an excellent time to practice strengthening his or her resilience—rather than focusing on the negative (the drug use itself), focus on developing a positive skill (healthy sleep habits) to help manage it. It's also another great reminder of how important sleep is to our overall health and sanity. Even if your kid isn't into drugs, getting a little extra sleep—and spending a little less time in front of a screen—is always a good idea. For us parents, too! **Time spent:** 5 minutes to talk about sleep habits, maybe 15 to install blackout shades, and who knows how long to debate about having removed the TV from the bedroom

Turn a nag into a snuggle—and then move away. One study looked at the mood states of 30 married couples and found that their negative moods and cortisol (a stress hormone) levels mirrored each other, especially at night, when they were in closer proximity. The one exception: When the marriage was a strong one, the spouses were protected—they did not necessarily absorb their spouses' bad moods. (In other words, they showed compassionate acceptance, but held to good boundaries.)

When your partner is having a bad day, make a conscious effort not to let it affect you. Ask if there's anything you can do, give an affectionate squeeze of the shoulders, and then let him or her be—don't try to offer advice or problem solve unless you're asked to. You may be trying to help, but unsolicited advice can feel like criticism when you're already down in the dumps. Just keep smiling and steer clear. **Time spent:** 1 minute for a good hug, which can really help in situations like this; repeat as necessary

Bring your best pal—but only one—to your next high-stress event. If, like many people, you struggle with giving public presentations, you may be incredibly hard on yourself and in the habit of saying awful things to yourself. With all of that self-criticism crashing around in your head, speaking in public (whether to the board of directors or to your PTA) can feel like a walk to the guillotine. But there are ways to manage that anxiety. In a study published in the journal *Psychosomatic Medicine*, 90 women gave a speech to an observer—either a stranger who seemed neutral, a stranger who seemed supportive, or a friend who seemed supportive. The study found that with the neutral listener, the speaker's systolic blood pressure rose by almost 23 points. When the stranger seemed supportive, it rose by almost 15 points. But when the friend listened, the speaker's blood pressure rose a mere 8 points, just more than a third of the impact of the neutral stranger.

Bring a supportive friend to your next speech and have her sit in the middle of the audience. Being able to see her and rest your eyes on her during the speech will help you manage your anxiety. It will also give you a visual picture for your next speech—

even if your friend can't attend, you can imagine her sitting out in the audience, giving you a mental high five. **Time spent:** 5 minutes to explain what you need to your best friend

Spend 5 minutes weeding your garden. Step out your back door for as little as 5 minutes and you can improve your mood, mental health, and self-esteem. A study done at the University of Essex looked at the experiences of 1,252 participants in the United Kingdom and revealed that the biggest effect was seen with just 5 minutes of activity done outside daily. Researchers were delighted with the findings, which marked the first time a study had found a "dose response" effect for something as broad and grand as the great outdoors. Kids felt the largest boost in self-esteem, so try to get them at least a short time in nature every day while they are little. The researchers found that the benefits increased if water was present—a koi pond or a frog habitat, perhaps. Or just get your hands in the dirt by starting an organic vegetable garden. If you go that route, you'll save money on produce by raising your own food, prevent greenhouse gas emissions—and delight in the experience of tasting a tomato fresh from the vine, still warm from the sun. When spring hits, stock up on those glorious days of sunshine and higher barometric pressure. Studies have proven that the more time you spend outside during springtime's warmer, brighter days, the better your mood and memory, and the more "broadened" mental flexibility and creativity you will have. (Get it while you can, because summer's hotter weather has the opposite effect!) **Time spent:** 5—minimum—sunbaked, glorious minutes outside a day

Talk with touch. Research on the therapeutic power of touch has revealed that when spouses, friends, and caregivers massage us, we feel more connected and content and less anxious. One study even showed that waitresses who touched their customers earned higher tips. Humans are cuddlebugs by nature—our endocrine systems are set up to release a cascade of positive pleasure chemicals when we receive a caring touch. But a new study has shown that we actually communicate way more in brief touches than we ever knew. Researchers at DePauw University in Greencastle, Indiana, paired up strangers and, after obscuring the participants' vision, asked one person to touch the other while imagining a specific emotion. The receiver of the touch then guessed what emotion was being communicated. When the researchers analyzed the data, they found that anger, fear, disgust, love, gratitude, and sympathy were decoded at frequencies that were greater than was attributable to chance and that there were minute, detectable physical differences in how each of these emotions was communicated.

Some people are more amenable to touching than others, but if you haven't been using this avenue of communication, try incorporating more small touches in your daily conversations—especially with people you love and with your own kids. Consider it another way to tell them how much they mean to you. Hold your son's or daughter's shoulders while you talk about the day, rub your spouse's back when you're in the elevator together, shake a person's hand in both of yours when you first meet—all of these extra moments of connection may not be consciously noted, but the loving feelings they convey will be absorbed and add another positive moment to your relationship together. Actions speak louder than words, and the act of touch speaks loudest of all. **Time spent:** anywhere from a second to an hour of snuggling on the couch watching TV or holding hands in the movie theater

Pick up the phone. Sometimes you just can't be with the people you love—even when you need them most. A study from the University of Wisconsin at Madison suggests that a phone call could be a very good second option—and, in some cases, may help calm you down as much as a well-timed hug. Researchers tested a group of 7- to 12-year-old girls after a public speaking challenge triggered their stress responses and significantly boosted their cortisol levels. Those girls whose mothers comforted them on the phone showed the same relaxation response as those who were hugged by their moms: Their levels of the soothing cuddle hormone oxytocin rose while the stress hormone cortisol drifted downward. The researchers said these results were further proof of women's "tend and befriend" tendencies under stress. They were also thrilled to discover that oxytocin—previously thought to be released only by close physical touch—could be released by phone. **Time spent:** 5 minutes on the phone with a supportive partner, parent, or friend might be all you need to regain your equilibrium during a rough time

Doctors

I'm so impatient and angry, and my husband and
I fight all the time. I've heard this isn't great
for my health. But what's really going on inside?

Everyone is slightly different, but here are the major ways the distressed mind can harm the body:

- Muscles tense.
- Heart rate increases.
- Blood pressure rises.
- Stress hormones go up.
- Blood is more likely to clot.
- The body doesn't process sugar very well.
- The immune system doesn't fight off infections as easily.

TWO SUGGESTIONS:

First, the moment you find yourself becoming impatient, stop to become aware of your thoughts and feelings. Also, take into account the exact objective facts about the situation in which you are becoming impatient. Be sure to separate out thoughts that are interpretations and observations about what you can see or hear that would hold up in a court of law.

Next, ask yourself 4 questions, focusing on the objective facts, not your interpretations.

1. Is this matter Important to me?
2. Is what I am thinking and feeling Appropriate to the facts of the situation?
3. Is this situation Modifiable in a positive way?
4. When I balance my needs and the needs of others, is taking action WORTH IT?

Telling yourself, "I A-M WORTH IT!"™ may help you to remember these questions and remind yourself why it's important to get a grip on your anger. If you get four "Yeses" to these questions, calm action is called for. Any "No" means it's better to change your reaction and chill out.

—*Virginia Williams, PhD, president of Williams LifeSkills, and* **Redford Williams, MD,**
professor of psychiatry, psychology, and medicine and director of the
Behavioral Medicine Research Center at Duke University Medical Center

Go to sleep an hour earlier. We talked about the importance of sleep in Chapter 3, Use Your Head. Not sleeping can certainly impact your brain's ability to learn, store memories, and even create new brain cells. But perhaps the most immediate impact sleep has is on your mood. Chronic sleep deprivation changes the way your brain handles serotonin, the neurotransmitter associated with pleasant, upbeat moods. Researchers believe that if our brains are consistently robbed of adequate sleep, the serotonin receptor system becomes desensitized and the brain is unable to process serotonin correctly. This desensitization is one of the mechanisms suspected of being at the heart of depression.

If your average sleep time doesn't come near the recommended 7 to 8 nightly hours, rather than sleeping later, try heading to bed earlier. If we fall asleep in the hours before midnight we're likely to have more non-REM sleep, and as a result to experience the phases of sleep associated with strengthening your immune system and letting your body do most of its repair work. **Time spent:** 60 glorious minutes of (early!) peaceful slumber

Play online with your partner. Dozens of studies done over many years have shown that people in happy, contented, mutually supportive relationships live longer. But these studies have also demonstrated that while positive relationships lead to health, negative relationships can lead to an early grave. In one study, couples who were the most hostile during a disagreement had the greatest increase in stress hormones and the greatest decrease in immune activity over the 24 hours that followed. Researchers believe that one way to head off these hostile habits is by learning as early as possible in your relationship how to fight fair, and a marriage counselor is a great person to help you with that. The best therapists will teach you and your partner how to share your feelings in an assertive, supportive way and how to negotiate with each other to get what you need.

So what do you do if you'd like to go to a marriage counselor but your husband or wife does not? Go online! Doctors at Baylor University in Waco, Texas, have created the Couple Conflict Consultant (www.pairbuilder.com), a free site that allows you and your partner to take interactive tests to help you zero in on your particular communication challenges. The program then gives you individualized tools that help you learn how to better communicate with each other and solve your conflicts. Your information is confidential and will help the scientists collect data for an ongoing research study. Win, win! **Time spent:** 5 minutes to create your profile and poke around the site—and then encourage your partner to do the same

Have a deep conversation. Be honest: Do you really care what the weather is like outside? We frequently exchange pleasantries with people—about the weather, the local sports team, the weekend. These moments of chatter are pleasant enough, but if we really want to be happy, we have to dig a little deeper.

A recent study published in *Psychological Science* found that people who spent more time locked in deep philosophical discussions were actually happier than those who skated along on the surface of conversational fodder. Researchers determined that those who were happiest enjoyed two times as much "deep" conversation and half as much small talk as those who were least happy. No surprise, the happiest people were outgoing and gregarious: They spent 25 percent less time alone and about 70 percent more time talking. But only 10 percent of those conversations were small talk, versus 28 percent for those who were the least happy.

Researchers say we tend to reveal ourselves in deeper conversations, which serves to draw us closer to the people we are sharing the thoughts with. And the more meaningful the conversation, the more closeness it creates. Go out for coffee with a person who is passionate about local politics. Or join a book club. Attend a meeting of the local township council or other community group. Get involved in any cause you feel passionate about—there are bound to be some like-minded folks to speak with. **Time spent:** 5 minutes to call your library and ask about book clubs, local author events, and other discussion groups that meet there

Put down your handheld. If you work at a computer, there is no end to the delights and distractions that can pull you away from your work. But before you beat yourself up for being undisciplined, you should know that novelty—like the "ping" of your e-mail notification or

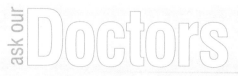

I've heard that optimists live longer—why
is that, and can I actually "teach" my kids
to be optimistic and happy?

The benefits reaped by optimists are numerous. Research shows us that compared to pessimistic
people, optimists are:

- More successful in school, at work, and in athletics
- Healthier and live longer
- More satisfied with their marriages
- Less likely to suffer from depression
- Less anxious

Who wouldn't want that list of benefits for their kids? There are three ways that kids learn to be
optimistic from their parents.

1. **Parental Affection:** Kids whose parents are caring and affectionate are more hopeful. Parental
   affection and care is—no surprises here—essential for kids to develop trust in the world. When
   kids have a secure base in their parents, they tend to believe that the world is a good place. In
   addition to fostering optimism, this allows them to take risks and explore—another way they
   learn to be optimistic.
2. **Taking Risks and Failing:** The ability to cope with challenge and frustration is critical for the

the lure of looking at *just one more* link before you start working—can be even more addictive

than cocaine. Recent research published in *Behavioral Neuroscience* found that the only thing

that could lure cocaine-addicted rats away from their drug were novel environments full of

interesting items. Now, your brain might require a bit more entertainment than a sock, a

scouring pad, or a balled-up newspaper, but the principle is the same.

Spare yourself the distraction. Keep your workspace neat and organized. Reduce piles of

paper and sticky notes on your monitor. Don't leave your e-mail on all day. Set 2 hours

development of optimism. Research shows that kids who are protected from failure and adversity are less likely to develop optimism. Why? When we make mistakes and learn from them we also learn that we can overcome the challenges that likely lie ahead. This makes us feel hopeful about the future.

3. **Modeling:** Pessimistic parents are more likely to have pessimistic children. More than modeling how optimistically or pessimistically we interpret events in our own lives, kids model how we interpret events in *their* lives. In other words, kids are more sensitive to the feedback they get from their parents than they are to their parents' explanations about their own life events. This means that when we criticize our children we make them more vulnerable to pessimism.

Ten-year-olds who are taught how to think and interpret the world optimistically are half as prone to depression when they later go through puberty. There are loads of ways to think optimistically:

- Identify the good that comes out of difficulty
- See the glass half full—point out what is good rather than what is bad even if both are present
- Choosing to trust: giving ourselves and others the benefit of the doubt rather than succumbing to self-doubt, blaming, or feeling offended

The research of famed psychologist Martin Seligman, who has studied optimism for decades, shows us that we definitely *can* teach our children to be optimistic and happy.

—***Christine Carter, PhD,*** *executive director of UC Berkeley's Greater Good Science Center and author of* Raising Happiness: 10 Simple Steps for More Joyful Kids and Happier Parents

aside, one in the morning and one in the afternoon, for receiving and answering e-mail. Prepare to be much more productive—and happier. **Time spent:** 15 seconds to turn off that e-mail notification!

Count each door you open. In two studies involving almost 300 people, Japanese researchers discovered that when participants were asked to count the number of kindnesses they showed to other people in the next week, the subjects' own feelings of happiness increased significantly.

Try it yourself—leave a more than generous tip for wait staff, open doors for people, pick up hats or scarves that are dropped, allow people to cut in line in front of you at the store. Jot them down every day. You may be encouraged to act kindly more often simply to tally a few more acts for your list. And that's perfectly okay, say the researchers, who concluded that, while happy people are kinder in the first place, they can become even happier, kinder, and more grateful simply by paying attention to how kind they are!

Another study found that "paying it forward"—showing a third person kindness after someone has been kind to you—truly does have an exponential effect, as much as tripling the "payout" down the line. You get to see the glee on someone else's face when you're kind, but you may not know how that kindness ripples into dozens and perhaps hundreds of other lives. **Time spent:** a few seconds—depending on the act—to be kind, but the effect could last a lifetime

Say a little prayer. One study published in the journal *Psychological Science* studied two groups of people—one whose members said a single prayer for the well-being of their spouses and another whose members simply described their spouses into a tape recorder. Afterward, the researchers measured forgiveness in all of the subjects and found that those who'd said the prayer were more likely to forget previous resentments and move on than those who hadn't. The researchers believe that this was because that initial prayer had moved each person's focus outward, away from him- or herself and onto other people. That group shifted from an interior focus to an exterior one, which opened up the possibility of forgiveness. Other research has suggested that forgiveness has powerful health benefits—so powerful, in fact, that it can reduce the risk of heart attack, slow the spread of cancer, and even prevent HIV from developing into AIDS—and a greatly improved immune system is something we all could use. And what relationship couldn't be improved with a little forgiveness? **Time spent:** a minute praying for the people you love (or simply meditating or thinking about them) to improve your own health in countless ways

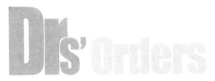

Drs' Orders

for a Healthy Emotional Life:
Surround Yourself with Positive People

Every day, researchers are learning more and more about the phenomenon of social contagion. We may believe we are the masters of our own domains—and, for the most part, we are—but the simple truth is that we are heavily influenced by everyone we come into contact with on a daily basis.

Researchers at Harvard and the University of California at San Diego have done some fascinating work looking at the impact of people's social circles on health outcomes like smoking, overweight, or depression. What they've found is that not only can one person influence another quite powerfully, one encounter can set off a chain reaction that spreads throughout a social network, impacting attitudes and behaviors sometimes even for years to come. Some of the most powerful effects are seen with happiness.

In one study, researchers determined that people's happiness can influence relationships to up to three degrees of separation (to the friends of your friends' friends). People who are surrounded by many happy people and those who are at the center of a network are more likely to become happy in the future. The researchers studied longitudinal statistical models and found that clusters of happiness result from happiness being spread, not just from people's tendency to associate with similar individuals.

Check this out: A friend who lives within a mile of you and becomes happy increases your chance of becoming happy by 25 percent. Having a happy spouse increases your chance of being happy by 8 percent; a happy sibling who lives within a mile has a 14 percent chance of making you happier. But who had by far the biggest effect? Your next-door neighbor. If he or she is happy, you have a 34 percent greater likelihood of being happy. And vice versa.

So, here's what we suggest: Smile and wave at the people in your neighborhood. Stop and talk when they walk by on the street. Get to know them by name, offer to take in their mail when they go on vacation. These things seem small, but they most definitely are not. (We'd like to see an antidepressant create 34 percent more happiness—it would be the best-selling drug on earth!)

And stay close: This study found that these positive network effects start to wane over time and geographic distance. Reach out, say hello—and keep saying hello. Your heart, and theirs (and their friend's heart, and their friend's friend's heart) will be the better for it. Can you imagine any better way to pay it forward?

Oh, Baby!

Perhaps nowhere else in human health is the miracle of life more evident than in our reproductive systems. Little girls come into this world with all the eggs they will ever have tucked away inside of them—they're born with the next generation already waiting in the wings. Many of them grow up to fall in love with men, who just happen to produce millions of eager-to-procreate sperm each day. Throw in some hormones, a little low lighting, and—*bam!*—the future of the human race is assured once again.

Mother Nature is like that—she likes to stack the deck in her own favor. Whether it's our intoxicating desire for sex, the cyclical nature of fertility, the ferocity of parental protectiveness, or even the gradual shutting down of the reproductive ability, Mother Nature wants everybody on earth to quit all their other shenanigans and focus on one thing and one thing only: making more people.

Fix It in 5
Protect Your Reproductive Health

1. Minimize stress.
2. Steer clear of endocrine disruptors.
3. Get 7 to 8 hours of good-quality sleep every night.
4. Manage your blood sugar effectively.
5. Feed yourself clean, whole organic foods.

Now, that doesn't mean we have to listen or that we don't have any free will. Not every person feels he or she must have children. In fact, in the modern world, we're seeing every flavor of personal choice when it comes to reproduction and child rearing. But regardless of what choices we make about what we do (or don't do) with the machinery, we all have the baby-making setup on board—and it influences an amazing number of different aspects of our lives.

Let's consider several ways in which our reproductive health impacts first our personal health and then the health of our offspring when we do get pregnant. Ultimately, you can use what nature gave you in any way you like—for pleasure and for procreation—and with a few 5-minute fixes here and there, you can make the entire life span of your reproductive system that much healthier.

A 5-Minute Tour of Your Reproductive System

Our bodies don't wait until we hit puberty to get sexual—we are sexual beings from birth, from the moment Dad's sperm bearing either an X or a Y chromosome plowed into Mom's egg. This chance meeting in a brief moment determines so much about our bodies for the rest of our lives.

We may like to believe that men and women are all just people—until they go to the bathroom or get busy between the sheets. But in every field of medicine, from cardiology to dermatology to neuroscience, researchers and clinicians are determining that men's and women's bodies are different at a very basic level: We think differently, smell differently, feel pain differently, handle stress differently. We want sex at different times. We form friendships (or don't) for different reasons.

Ultimately, if you do decide you want to have kids, the best gift you can give them is to be healthy yourself, and to have a healthy partner. And our choices throughout life provide the critical foundation for our kids' longevity long before they're even conceived. Luckily for all of us, these steps benefit aspiring parents and nonparents alike. Sexual health is a gift that keeps on giving, no matter who's on the receiving end: ourselves, our partners, or our kids.

Mama Mia

The reproductive system is a complex system that involves organs, hormones, eggs, and sperm—and some luck. We'll get to the guys in a bit—but just as in men, most of a woman's reproductive machinery is located in the pelvis. The outside covering of the female reproductive organs, called the vulva, protects the entrance to the womb and the urine transport system called the urethra. You might call them the curtains hiding the main stage, the vagina.

The vagina is a muscular canal that leads to the womb, or uterus. The vagina is kind of like a tunnel the sperm travels through to make its way to the egg. It's also the route the baby takes in the opposite direction to enter the world, after the uterine walls contract to push the baby out, almost like squeezing a tube of toothpaste, which is actually the cramping feeling you get when the uterus is contracting to get all the menstrual blood out. Prostaglandins, those hormonelike substances involved in pain and inflammation, can set off those uterine muscle contractions—and the more prostaglandins you have, the more severe menstrual cramps you'll get, too.

The neck of the uterus, the cervix, connects the uterus to the vagina. The cervix is a ring of connective tissue covered with a very thin layer of muscle whose opening expands to allow a baby to pass through. If you're pregnant, get ready for the shock of your life when your ob-gyn or midwife shows you that gauge of what 2 centimeters looks like versus 10—the 10 that you'll stretch when it's time to give birth.

But in the grand scheme of a woman's lifetime, unless you have a big family, all that baby-making machinery may only get put to nature's intended purpose a small handful of times—if ever. Luckily for all women, there's this activity, called S-E-X, during which a gal and her partner can put to use many fun little features of the female reproductive system. Chief among these is the small, sensitive organ of erectile tissue tucked away behind the vulva, called the clitoris. And while the female version of this organ seems exclusively built for pleasure, the guys' version—the penis—is called upon to be quite the biological multitasker.

What's That, Daddy?

The male system boasts the penis, testicles, and prostate gland (and we do mean "boast"). The testicles are glands that make and house the sperm, and they hang outside the body in the scrotum, a sac that acts like a thermostat by tightening up to bring the testicles close to the body to keep sperm warm when temperatures get cold and expanding away from the body when it gets hot out. This one action enables the testicles to keep the sperm in a healthy, temperate climate.

Those little guys cannot travel on their own, so sperm need to be mixed with a fluid called

DOCTOR, DOCTOR, GIMME THE NEWS: HIV VACCINE

In the early days of the HIV/AIDS epidemic, the virus primarily affected the gay male population in this country, leading many to believe that it was a gay disease. Fast-forward to 2010, and one-quarter of new HIV/AIDS diagnoses are in women. HIV/AIDS is the leading cause of death among black women ages 25 to 34 in this country. And while condoms have been shown to effectively prevent the spread of HIV, people continue to have unprotected sex, and some women, especially in developing countries, aren't able to refuse to have sex with a man even if he isn't wearing a condom. But new research may lead to a new method of HIV protection that will allow women to arm themselves against the virus.

Research published in the *Journal of Biological Chemistry* reported that a protein called BanLec that is derived from bananas may help prevent the transmission of HIV. In laboratory tests, BanLec effectively thwarted infection with HIV by attaching itself to a particular type of sugar that the virus has a high concentration of. HIV is then unable to attach to and infect human cells. "BanLec is made from lectins, which are proteins in plants that are capable of binding to sugars," says David Markovitz, MD, who is researching the chemical along with a team of scientists at the University of Michigan at Ann Arbor. "The coat of the HIV virus is rich in sugar, which is why sugar-binding lectins were thought to be a good candidate." Dr. Markovitz and his team are hoping to incorporate BanLec into a gel and test its efficacy outside the lab. "One of the reasons that an HIV vaccine has been slow in coming is that the virus mutates, making it difficult to develop a drug," says Dr. Markovitz. "What is amazing about BanLec is its ability to work on various types of the HIV, which makes it more difficult for HIV to become resistant." But don't think that eating bananas will protect you from HIV—BanLec is a chemical that has been carefully isolated and produced. We'll all have to wait and see whether this promising vaccine actually hits the market in the future.

semen, which is manufactured in the seminal vesicles and prostate and travels through a tube called the vas deferens. The sperm leave the testicles via the vas deferens to meet up with the semen, and that happy, sperm-filled fluid is sent to the penis. The urethra, a channel inside the penis, is like a train track that routes either semen or urine from the body depending on which track is open.

Let Me Tell You 'bout the Birds and the Bees

These happy little glands, organs, and hormones are delighted to get the reproductive system cracking in puberty, which begins at about ages 8 to 13 for girls and 10 to 15 for boys. The pituitary gland begins to release certain hormones that send the signal for boys to begin producing testosterone and girls to begin producing estrogen. With the increase in testosterone, boys begin the invisible process of sperm production, along with the incredibly noticeable voice deepening and hair growth on their face, underarms, and genitals.

In girls, the ovaries produce estrogen, which primes them to eventually start pumping out those eggs and dropping them into the fallopian tubes for the initial cycle of menstruation, or menarche. But before that big day ever happens, many visible changes begin, starting first with pubic hair growth and then breast bud development. Stunned parents watch as both girls and boys experience growth spurts and weight gain more dramatic than anything they've seen since their babies were born. Sadly, along with this growth spurt comes a spurt in body odor and acne. Welcome to puberty!

Trouble in Babyland

While baby making can be quite simple, sometimes a number of problems present themselves: Damaged sperm, old eggs, or functional problems with the sexual organs can all lead to fertility problems. One in six couples has trouble getting pregnant when they want to, but modern science has managed to overcome many of the factors that lead to infertility, and couples who would never have had children a century ago are starting families. For example, in vitro fertilization allows eggs and sperm to be brought together in a petri dish. The fertilized eggs are then transferred to the woman's uterus, where she may be able to success-fully carry the fetus or fetuses to term. Doctors often implant multiple embryos in the uterus, and if they all survive, the woman ends up with more than one baby. Other techniques include injecting sperm directly into a fallopian tube, extracting sperm directly from a testicle, and administering certain drugs that increase ovulation. The method used is deter-mined by the cause of the infertility.

We're Pregnant—Now What?

Making babies is one of the most fun things in the world—and Mother Nature likes it that way. She needs to make sure we keep doing it! The amazingly complex process goes like this:

During ovulation, the eggs travel from the ovaries into the fallopian tubes to await the arrival of sperm. If sperm are delivered to the vagina during this time, one or more eager little go-getter sperm cells, fighting like hell to beat out the competitors, will head a little farther out than the rest and meet the egg in the fallopian tube. If no sperm cells enter the fallopian tubes, the lonely egg will dry up and be disposed of along with blood and tissues that were lining the uterus to prepare it for the implantation that didn't happen. This is that monthly delight called menstruation.

Seems pretty straightforward, no? But not all sperm cells can make the journey success-fully. Sperm needs to have three things going for it to accomplish its mission: quality, quantity, and motility. A sperm cell has to be a certain shape—an oval head with a long tail. There also must be millions of sperm in each batch of semen ejaculated from the penis. If there are fewer than 20 million sperm, a couple might experience problems becoming pregnant. Mind-boggling! The clincher: The sperm cells need to be strong swimmers to get to the eggs and push their way inside to fertilize them. When all of these conditions come together, *whew!* you're in the baby-making business.

Welcoming Menopause

Fast-forward through your baby-making years, and you're at the other side before you know it. Eventually, after some years of hormonal ups and downs, bad moods, and a lot of chocolate, the

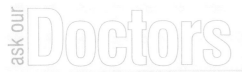

How do I know whether I need genetic testing or counseling before I get pregnant?

Dr. Lisa says . . .

Many couples don't have to include genetic counseling or tests in their prepregnancy planning. But if you're at a higher than normal risk for having an inherited disease, testing could bring you peace of mind if the results reveal that you're not a carrier. And if you are, having the information can help you and your partner make informed decisions about proceeding with your plans to become pregnant, as well as preparing for what's involved in caring for a child who may have special medical needs.

Your first step? Talk with your gynecologist or family doctor. He or she may recommend that you meet with a genetic counselor to help you decide whether you and your partner should be tested. It may be recommended if you are:

- African American and could pass sickle-cell anemia on to your children
- Of Southeast Asian or Mediterranean descent and could pass on a severe type of anemia called thalassemia
- Of Eastern European Jewish descent and could be a carrier of Tay-Sachs or Canavan disease, both of which can be fatal in early childhood
- From a family with a history of inherited disorders such as cystic fibrosis, hemophilia, or muscular dystrophy, or if you have relatives with birth defects or severe developmental problems
- A woman who has had several miscarriages
- A woman who is over age 35

A test can't, in most cases, tell you with certainty whether your child would inherit a genetic condition, but the results can help a genetic counselor estimate the odds.

babes are out of the nest or soon to be, and your reproductive ability comes to a gradual, usually welcome halt. Ovaries winnow down their production of estrogen and progesterone beginning at about age 30, which means that fewer eggs are prepared each month until eventually that process (and menstruation) stops completely—usually when you are in your fifties.

I keep hearing conflicting things about
prostate exams. What's the story—should I get one or not?

Dr. Travis says . . .

That depends! (You knew I was going to say that, didn't you?)

A prostate exam is a test that screens for prostate cancer. The goal is to detect cancer early, when treatment will be most successful. The most common prostate exam is the digital rectal exam, in which the doctor inserts his or her gloved, lubricated finger into the rectum to blindly feel the prostate gland and surrounding tissues.

The Cleveland Clinic recommends that all men have an annual prostate exam beginning at age 45, and they suggest that the following folks also have a particular blood test annually:

- All men beginning at age 50
- African American men beginning at age 40
- Men with a family history of prostate cancer beginning at age 45 (or younger, if it's recommended by a doctor)

Men may also experience some fertility issues as they age. Diseases like cancer, diabetes, and heart disease can damage the muscles and tissues needed for erections or to manufacture sperm. Also, all guys go through a small natural decline in testosterone levels—after age 40, testosterone dips by about 1 to 2 percent per year. Only a small percentage of men truly have low testosterone levels, though; even by age 75, only 30 percent have clinically low levels of testosterone. But if you take care to keep blood flowing to all of your tissues and organs by exercising and eating right for a few decades, you can maintain a good degree of sexual prowess. The *American Journal of Cardiology* found that guys who have sex two or three times a week have 45 percent less heart disease than those who have sex less than once a month. No doubt about it—their partners benefit, too.

The controversial part of that is the blood test, which measures prostate-specific antigen (PSA), a substance produced by the prostate gland. An elevated PSA level may indicate prostate cancer or a noncancerous condition such as prostatitis, which is inflammation of the gland usually caused by an infection, or benign prostatic hyperplasia, which is often called an enlarged prostate.

Now, the risk of prostate cancer is not that small: The American Cancer Society says as many as 192,000 cases are diagnosed every year. However, we're seeing more and more evidence that PSA screening results are not that precise and are resulting in unnecessary treatment—which, in some cases, can be more debilitating than the relatively mild abnormalities detected. (Indeed, the American Cancer Society does not currently recommend routine prostate cancer screening.)

Treatment of prostate cancer depends on how old and how healthy you are, how aggressive the cancer is (reported as a Gleason score), and the stage of the cancer (meaning whether and where it has spread to other parts of the body). Treatment options for prostate cancer include active surveillance, hormone therapy, cryosurgery, various types of radiation therapy, open pros-tatectomy, robot-assisted laparoscopic prostatectomy, and chemotherapy. Only after having a careful evaluation performed by and discussion with a physician specializing in prostate cancer should you decide on a course of therapy. The side effects of some treatments can be serious, like incontinence and impotence.

Bottom line: Talk to your doctor to see if your family or personal history warrants testing now, or if you can hold off for a while.

5-Minute Fixes
for a Lifetime of Men's Sexual Health

If there's one part of the body that guys don't even want to dream they might have problems with, it's that whole nether region. Luckily, as body systems go, the penis and scrotum are pretty low maintenance. (After all, most guys like to, ahem, rotate the tires and get that oil changed as often as possible.) Let's talk about some routine maintenance measures guys can do in 5 minutes or less to help protect the engine (and its cylinders) for years to come.

Snack your way to good sex. It's true! Certain foods can have actions in the body that either stimulate certain sex hormones or increase blood flow—both of which definitely add spice in the bedroom. Try a couple of these for better sex tonight.

> **Avocados:** Contain folic acid and vitamin B$_6$, both of which stimulate the thyroid and spur the creation of male and female hormones. Holy guacamole.

> **Capsaicin:** Found in hot peppers, capsaicin stimulates your natural endorphins, and it can also help you burn fat while you get randy. Also found in some lubricants—can you say "hot"?—it is effective for women, too.

> **Celery:** Celery is chock-full of androsterone, a male pheromone that comes out in your sweat, and though it isn't consciously smelled, it drives women crazy.

Time spent: 5 minutes to pick one of these snacks and enjoy their "benefits" with your partner

Stack it up. If you're looking to increase your overall virility, your muscles are your body's best testosterone producer—though doing a "12-ounce curl" isn't the answer. The trick is to really push yourself while you're working out. One Finnish study found that "forced repetitions" of resistance exercise—doing as many reps as possible with the heaviest weights and then being assisted in completing the set—resulted in significant rises in serum testosterone, free testosterone, cortisol, and growth hormone concentrations. The researchers attributed the hormonal boost to the intensity of the exercise. Another study found that men who lifted weights regularly had as much as 49 percent more free testosterone than those who didn't.

Work with a trainer to develop the best program for your current fitness level, and definitely use a spotter at the gym if you're going for broke and hefting the heaviest weight loads. **Time spent:** 30 minutes twice a week

We're going to try to get pregnant soon, and I'm a little nervous about my boys down there. Is there anything I can do to boost my sperm count?

Dr. Lisa says . . .

Low sperm count may be an issue for a third to a half of all couples struggling with infertility. A fertility specialist can analyze your sperm for quantity and to see if they're healthy and good swimmers. But these do-it-yourself steps can help, too.

Keep 'em cool. Sperm are produced in a man's testicles. The ideal conditions for a bumper crop: Temperatures several degrees below the body's core temperature. Wearing tight briefs or tight pants can heat things up enough to lower your sperm count. So can soaking in a hot tub, hanging out in a sauna, and wearing tight workout shorts. Opt for boxer shorts and avoid overheating.

Kick the butts. Smoking cigarettes can reduce sperm count.

Drink moderately. Stick with a two-drinks-a day limit. Consuming more alcohol than that can torpedo sperm production.

Stay slim and trim. Extra pounds may interfere with a man's ability to produce lots of healthy sperm. The cause? It could be out-of-balance hormones, extra body heat, or the effects of a high-calorie diet and lack of exercise.

Enjoy regular sex. Experts used to say that abstaining for a few days before trying to become pregnant built up a man's sperm reserves. But a recent Australian study finds that daily sex improves sperm quality and boosts motility—sperm's ability to swim.

Avoid recreational drugs. There are plenty of good reasons to steer clear of marijuana, cocaine, and anabolic steroids used for bodybuilding, and you can add protecting sperm to the list. All reduce sperm count significantly.

5-Minute Fixes

for a Lifetime of Women's Sexual Health

Most of a woman's routine medical care as an adult involves her reproductive organs. Long before the average woman has a regular yearly checkup with a primary care physician, she goes for her "annual exam"—a Pap test at the gynecologist's office. After the age of 40, this annual going-over may also include a mammogram of her breasts, an experience whose discomfort is caused by a surreal level of flesh squashing.

Because of the ever-changing nature of menstrual cycles, women's sexual health needs may change every few years—or even every few months. Overall it's a matter of supporting our smart bodies as they follow those internal rhythms that often function like clockwork. When we have those moments when the hormones get wild—before and after periods, childbirth, and menopause—a few well-timed 5-minute fixes can get us back on a smooth and steady course once again.

Don't get flooded. Dr. Lisa calls menstrual fluid a vital sign for women. If your periods are so heavy that you are soaking through a tampon, pad, and your clothes, you could have a condition called menorrhagia. If there are clots, it's called clotting, and if it comes fast and thin, it could be something called flooding. Caused by everything from early perimenopause to uterine fibroids and endometrial problems, these types of bleeds are not just annoying, they can require blood transfusions or even become life-threatening. Repeated bleeds could require a surgical intervention, possibly even a hysterectomy.

How do you know if you have flooding? If you go through a super tampon or a super pad every hour, or if you feel light-headed all the time, you need to get it checked out. You may be anemic—many women become anemic due to heavy periods—and could benefit from taking birth control, progesterone, or iron supplements. While you're at the doctor's,

My wife and I are trying erectile dysfunction
drugs for the first time. What do I do if I have
an erection that lasts for more than 4 hours?

Dr. Travis says . . .

First of all, don't ruin what should be a pleasurable experience by worrying! Four-hour
erections are actually quite rare. But while this uncommon side effect of Viagra (sildenafil), Cialis (tadalafil), or Levitra (vardenafil) is often joked about, it's actually a very serious,
painful condition called priapism. When you experience priapism, you are not aroused;
your erection doesn't go away even if you have already ejaculated. Instead, a circulation
malfunction traps blood in the penis, cutting off the fresh oxygen supply to the
tissues—and potentially leaving you with permanent tissue damage.

Whatever you do, do not ignore this condition—one of the most common long-term
effects is erectile dysfunction. If you're treated within 24 hours, you have a less than 10
percent chance of being left with any long-term problems. But if you wait a week or more,
your risk of impotence jumps to 78 percent. So if it happens, get to the ER, stat.

have your blood tested. You might be a good candidate for birth control pills.

Here's the lowdown on clots: An occasional clot the size of a marble or smaller is totally
normal. But anything bigger than that indicates a problem, and you must go see the doctor.
You may have fibroids or cervical polyps, clotting problems, unusual vaginal discharge, or
cervical infection or inflammation. Or, it could be an indication of cancer (depending on your
age). You might also have been pregnant and be having a miscarriage.

Overall, your flow should be a nice, steady stream, with not too much clotting. Look for
these colors:

Brownish to red: Totally normal. These are the most common colors, representing mostly the endometrial lining of the uterus, plus vaginal fluids and cervical mucus.

Dark brown: Most likely just old blood

Bright red and constant: If the bleeding is copious and not clotting, it could mean you're flooding. Make an appointment right away. If you start to feel light-headed or you're scared by the large quantity of your flow, have someone take you to the emergency room.

All this talk of heavy flow said, the flipside—less frequent periods—may also be a concern. Play it safe: If your periods are starting to get farther and farther apart—and especially if you only have two or three periods a year—please see your doctor. **Time spent:** If it's not an emergency, take 5 minutes to give your gynecologist a call to set up an appointment—don't wait!

tampon or sanitary pad every 1 to 2 hours—you have bleeding between periods, or you have bleeding after menopause.

Pain during sex: Pain in your vagina during intercourse may be a sign of vaginal dryness due to shifting hormones around the time of menopause. A water-soluble lubricant can help; so can more foreplay to stimulate natural lubrication.

See your doctor if: You have any smelly or unusually colored vaginal discharge, have muscle spasms that make intercourse difficult or impossible, or feel pain deeper in your vagina or abdomen. This could be a sign of endometriosis, pelvic inflammatory disease, ovarian cysts, or other conditions. Painful intercourse may also be a symptom of chlamydia or gonorrhea, so be sure to see your doctor and get tested.

Breast pain and tenderness: Having some tenderness is normal around the time of your period or in the second half of your cycle, after you ovulate. You may feel a burning, itching, or aching pain if you have fibrocystic breasts, in which small, harmless cysts can swell or become tender usually around the time of menstruation.

See your doctor if: You have discharge from your nipples or you notice a lump that's new or different.

Afraid to jump up and down and laugh at the same time? Approximately 13 million Americans (85 percent of them women) experience urinary incontinence, or loss of bladder control, so it's no surprise that we get a *lot* of viewer mail about this potentially embarrassing condition. Urinary incontinence has two major subtypes: stress and urge.

Stress Incontinence: Stress incontinence occurs when the sphincter muscle of the bladder is weak, resulting in involuntary loss of urine when stress (pressure) is exerted. "Stress" can be a cough, sneeze, laugh, or physical activity. Women who have experienced pregnancy, childbirth, or menopause often develop stress incontinence due to the physical changes in their bodies. Treatments depend on the underlying condition and include medication, biofeedback and pelvic floor muscle training (sometimes called Kegel exercises), surgery, and behavioral changes like going to the bathroom a bit more frequently.

Urge Incontinence: Urge incontinence occurs when the bladder muscles spasm, and it is also referred to as overactive bladder. A person will experience an intense, sudden urge to urinate and often will not make it to the toilet in time. Urge incontinence can result from a variety of health problems such as a current urinary tract infection, nervous system damage, and bowel problems. Treatments depend on the underlying condition and include medication, bladder retraining (by peeing often to keep bladder nearly empty and then gradually retraining it to hold urine), and surgery.

Give your gynecologist a call to see what remedies are best for you. But do something! Many women stop doing aerobic exercise or avoid wearing certain clothing because they're terrified of wetting themselves in public. That's no way to live—not when there are so many effective alternatives. Make a call. **Time spent:** 1 minute to jump, 2 minutes to change your panties, and 5 minutes to call for an appointment

Change your underwear. We'll assume you changed your underwear after your incontinence experiment—that's not what we're talking about here. Did you know that about 20 percent of women will get at least one bladder infection in their lives? When you have one, you feel pressure in the pelvis and achiness in your lower abdomen, have a slight fever, and need to urinate frequently even though it hurts. The best ways to prevent these infections are to urinate regularly and empty your bladder completely every time you do. Also, wearing cotton underwear and loose clothing can help keep that area cool and dry, which helps since bacteria thrive in warm, damp places. Drink plenty of liquids, including cranberry juice, which helps keep bacteria from attaching to the bladder. Stay away from drinks that are known to irritate the bladder, such as coffee and alcohol. If you find yourself with a bladder infection, call your doctor, because it can lead to a serious kidney infection. **Time spent:** 5 minutes at the store picking out some cute cotton undies and 30 seconds a day to put them on

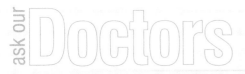

I seem to keep getting urinary tract infections—how can I avoid them? Are there any natural ways to treat them?

Urinary tract infections are very common and account for a large number of doctor visits. Here are some natural ways of treating and preventing urinary tract infections:

Drink cranberry juice and take vitamin C supplements, both of which help to acidify the urine and get rid of harmful bacteria which are the culprits of the infection.

Drink plenty of water to flush the urinary tract of toxins and bacteria—in addition, water keeps us hydrated to fight infections off faster.

Don't wait too long! Another important key of preventing urinary tract infections—which may be difficult for a woman—is, when you have to urinate, don't hold it. Holding it till you finish the tasks of day allows bacteria to grow into a full-blown infection of the urinary tract.

Wipe well—when you are done having a bowel movement it is imperative you wipe from front to back to avoid bacteria being spread from the anus to the urethra.

This last one is very important: Urinate before and after sexual intercourse to keep bacteria from transferring to the urethra and creating a breeding ground for urinary tract infections.

These few simple, natural ways can go a long way of preventing urinary tract infections.

—**Nancy Georgekutty, MD,** *a primary care physician with the Mansfield Medical Group at Methodist Mansfield Medical Center in Dallas, Texas*

Don't skimp on the chocolate-covered pretzels. When you have PMS, your hormones may make you crave either salty or very sweet foods. You may feel irritable and bloated and have sore breasts. PMS can be really debilitating depending on its severity, and no walk in the park even on an easy day. Although it may seem somewhat counterintuitive to a die-hard high protein fan, carbs can be your friend: carbohydrates can increase the amount of the neurotransmitter serotonin in your brain, which will increase your sense of well-being. Eating complex carbohydrates—whole grains and vegetables—is the healthiest way to get that serotonin increase. Calcium helps lessen bloating, so also go for milk, yogurt, or sardines. Right before you menstruate, be careful to avoid things that are estrogenic, like alcohol and soy. And if things get really bad, indulge yourself with a handful of dopamine-increasing, carbohydrate-packed chocolate-covered pretzels to give your poor, overtired PMS-suffering brain the equivalent of a warm bath. **Time spent:** 5 minutes in the store stocking up and 5 minutes to tear into them when the time is right

Check out another woman's breasts. No, we mean it. So many women don't have a clue about how to do a breast self-exam. They're worried that they won't do it "right," so they don't even try. If this sounds like you, go to YouTube and just type in "self breast exam." You'll be able to see exactly how to give yourself the exam, which is helpful if the only person to ever do one on you is your ob-gyn.

Another option is the Mark for Life T-shirt (www.markforlife.com) that Dr. Lisa featured on the show last year. These T-shirts have concentric circles over the breasts and show the exact pattern to follow to examine your breasts thoroughly. If you find something worrisome, you can mark its location with a permanent marker on the T-shirt and then bring it to your doctor as a kind of road map to the trouble spot.

Here are a few brief reminders about how to perform these exams. Don't worry about doing it perfectly—no one's grading you. Just do it!

Lying on your back:

- Starting near your armpit, move your fingers around the breast in one direction, spiraling in until you're at your nipple.
- Or, move your fingers up and down in straight lines that gradually work their way over to the other side of your breast.

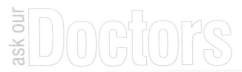
ask our **Doctors**

```
I sometimes get really turned on during
my period. Is that weird?
```

Dr. Lisa says . . .

I get this question all the time! The thing is, your period can be a really sexy time. Through-out your cycle, your hormone levels go up and down, and your libido rises and falls in response.

Your blood level of estrogen goes up around the time of ovulation, so a lot of women typically get more sexually aroused around then—which makes sense, from an evolution-ary standpoint, because that's when you're the most fertile.

During your period, it's all about testosterone. Women produce testosterone in their ovaries and their adrenal glands, and its level goes up and down during your period. Add in the fact that, due to fluctuating levels of estrogen and progesterone, there's a lot of blood rushing down there, making you slightly engorged and certainly well lubricated. If your partner is into it, this is actually a great time to have sex because you're feeling womanly, estrogen has stimulated your breasts, and you are more sensitive to sexual stimulation.

I say just go with it! A lot of people may not want to have sex during the woman's period because it's messy. But orgasm can be a great cramp reliever!

Then, standing in front of the mirror, look at both breasts:

- Are they lopsided? (Or if they always were, are they more so than usual?)
- Is there any unusual puckering?
- Is there any discharge from the nipple?
- Do you see any changes in the contour of the breast?

Again, don't stress about doing it "right"; this is not a recipe. The ultimate goal is to "get to know" your breasts after a few months. And that's the best defense against missing any changes. **Time spent:** 5 well-spent minutes each month

5-Minute Fixes
for a Healthy Pregnancy

You can give your baby the best start by feeding yourself well, getting enough rest, keeping a lid on stress, and staying positive. But aside from that, you don't have much input. Your body does all the work, whether you're thinking about being a good mommy or not. That certainly won't be the case once the child's born, so try not to stress too much about pregnancy and enjoy being so incredibly productive without lifting an extra finger! After the baby is born, well that's another story . . . that's when the heavy lifting begins.

For now, try a few of these 5-minute fixes to help yourself relax and enjoy both your pregnancy and being the center of attention—because soon enough, you'll be upstaged by a bald little butterball. And remember, moms and babies need regular pre- and postnatal visits to stay healthy.

Eat for 1.1 instead of for 2. Contrary to that old wives' tale, you don't need to—and shouldn't—eat for two when you're pregnant. If they were at a healthy weight when they conceived, pregnant moms actually only need about 10 percent more calories during pregnancy. Work with your doctor to determine the optimum number of calories to get you to these recommended weight ranges:

- If your starting weight was normal (BMI of 18.5 to 24.9), you should gain 25 to 35 lbs
- If your starting weight was lower than normal (BMI lower than 18.5), you should gain 35 to 40 lbs
- If your starting weight was higher than normal (BMI higher than 25), you should gain 15 to 20 lbs

Heck, following orders might not even be that hard to do: The bonus benefit of sticking to a strict regimen when you're pregnant is that the typical woman finds it much easier to follow the doctor's orders because she's more concerned about any risks to her child than to

How do I know if I'm gaining too much weight during my pregnancy? Is it terrible if I don't really care?

Dr. Lisa says . . .

If you were at a healthy, normal weight when you conceived (with a BMI between 18.5 and 24.9), putting on 25 to 35 pounds during your pregnancy is considered healthy. It means you're eating and drinking enough to supply the raw materials for your growing baby and also for your growing uterus and breasts, for your own increased blood supply, and for the extra body fat you store up to help support breastfeeding.

But the right amount of gain for you may be higher or lower; for example, putting on up to 40 pounds may be better if you started out your pregnancy underweight; as little as 20 to 25 pounds may be recommended if you were obese. (Work with your doctor to be sure you're getting enough nutrients to nourish your baby.)

Don't worry if you're a little bit above or below these levels, or if you have one or two growth spurts when you gain several pounds quickly. But it's important to know that gaining extra weight could raise your risk for developing gestational diabetes or a dangerous form of high blood pressure called preeclampsia during your pregnancy—conditions your doctor will check for throughout. Gaining extra weight could also create a bigger baby, increasing the chances you'll need a Caesarean. C-sections are becoming more common—32 percent of babies in the US are now delivered that way. But in case you're tempted to go that route by elective C-section, remember—the procedure still carries risks, like any surgery.

Experts say "eating for two" doesn't really mean doubling up on portions and calories. It takes about 300 extra calories of healthy foods per day to give your growing baby what he or she needs—that's the amount in a glass of fat-free milk paired with half of a peanut butter and jelly sandwich.

herself. **Time spent:** 5 minutes to discuss and determine the best calorie limit with your doctor, and 2 minutes at every meal to eyeball portions and control calories

Put down the fork and head for the door. Fewer than one in four pregnant women gets as much exercise as she needs. Adhering to a regular exercise program not only protects the baby from harm, it helps you. Dragging your partner or a friend out on a brisk 10-minute walk after every lunch and dinner can help you manage your body's postprandial (after eating) insulin response better than if you stay at the kitchen table chatting. Aerobic exercise of any kind immediately helps your body process insulin better. Walks count, sure, and so do vacuuming, dancing around the living room, walking the stairs at the baseball stadium . . . String together enough of these postmeal insulin-management moments to make up the minimum suggested time—30 minutes a day—and you just might baby-step yourself away from diabetes risk in the years to come. **Time spent:** 30 minutes a day (10 minutes after lunch and dinner, plus two 5-minute walks), 5 days a week

Mom-to-be, meet your husband, the masseur. One study done at the University of Miami medical school found that when pregnant moms were down in the dumps, getting massages from their partners really turned their moods around. Women with prenatal depression—depression before the birth instead of after the birth, which is more common—received massages twice a week from their partners beginning at 20 weeks' gestation and continuing until the end of their pregnancies. When compared with the control group, these women reported lower levels of leg pain, back pain, sadness, anxiety, and anger. Surprisingly, their partners also reported fewer depressed moods as well as less anger and anxiety. When asked about their relationships, both the husbands and the wives reported improvements there as well. Buy some nice lotion and let him get to work. Bonus: It just might lead to more than a massage, which is great for both of you. **Time spent:** 20 minutes a day for two 10-minute massages—or as often as your partner would like!

Become a flossing queen. Without regular flossing, plaque and bacteria can build up on teeth and cause gingivitis, which is inflammation of the gums. Gingivitis can progress to periodontitis, which leads to the gradual loss of the bone and tissues that support the teeth. In addition, the bacteria involved are systemic, which means that they circulate throughout the bloodstream and can cause more serious health problems, such as cardiovascular disease. In

```
I'm pregnant—how come I feel like such an
idiot? Is there really such a thing as "momnesia"?
```

Dr. Lisa says . . .

Many of my patients talk about "mommy brain," that brain-dead feeling you have during pregnancy and early parenthood. But I want to reassure you that if there is such a thing, it certainly is not a long-lasting condition. In fact, one recent animal study suggests that our brains might actually get stronger after we give birth. Researchers found that the brains of rats that had had more than one litter were more receptive to estrogen later in life. Estrogen is a key element in the work of the brain, helping the neural signal system and directing blood to parts of the brain that are more active.

Another recent study gave us an additional hint about what might be going on here. Researchers at the University of British Columbia in Vancouver did a study on pregnant women and found that they performed just as well as nonpregnant women on tests of memory when they were in the lab, but did not do as well outside of the lab setting. The researchers of the unpublished study concluded that while you're pregnant, it's likely you are experiencing the scatterbrained feeling that comes when your attention is divided among too many things at once.

Also, don't forget that once your baby's born, in the early stages, before he or she settles into a more mature circadian rhythm, you may not be sleeping for more than an hour or two at a time—which means that you may not get to complete a full 90-minute sleep cycle. So you're frequently disrupted from getting to your non-REM restorative sleep.

But rest assured—all of the new feelings, emotions, and thoughts you're experiencing are stimulating tremendous growth in your brain. If anything, a "mommy brain" is a much stronger, more resilient brain.

women who are pregnant, these bacteria can pass through the placenta and increase the chances of preterm birth by an astonishing 700 percent.

Some people floss after every meal; that's fine, but not necessary. Floss once a day, before bed. If you don't like the feeling of floss on your fingers, invest in a bag of those disposable plastic flossers.

Plaque is like an ongoing infection that the body must fight. After years of this, the immune system gets worn down and is at greater risk for serious diseases like cancer, diabetes, and pneumonia. **Time spent:** 3 minutes to floss once or twice a day

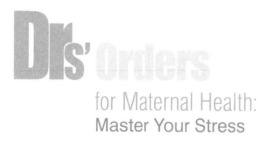

Drs' Orders
for Maternal Health:
Master Your Stress

Having a baby can be a joyous event, but it can also bring a lot of stress into your life. Sometimes just being pregnant is stressful—you don't want your boss to find out, or you're worried about what it will do to your relationship, or you're afraid money's too tight to feed another mouth. But the kindest thing we can do for ourselves and for our children is to learn to let the stress go.

Studies abound that prove that stress is a major issue for expectant moms. Not only does it lower your quality of life, it may directly impact the wiring of your child's brain. In one study, moms who were emotionally frazzled (by everyday hassles, depression, or anxiety) as well as biochemically frazzled (by cortisol and epinephrine) had proportionally smaller babies. Bottom line: You need to take time for yourself—for yourself and for your babe.

Besides angling for that twice-daily massage, see how many other self-nurturing treats you can add to each day:

- Rub thick skin cream on your feet and slip on some plush socks for moisturizing while you read or watch something you love.

- Attend a pregnancy yoga class to learn a few relaxing poses that will help you manage your anxiety about the birth. You may even be able to use some of them during the birth itself!

- To give yourself time to relax after the birth, ask your partner or mom (or a friend whose taste you trust) to buy the thank-you note cards now so you'll have them ready to go once the onslaught of gifts begins.

- Send out a preemptive group e-mail to friends and family: "Thank you so much for your support over these months. We're so excited that he's almost here. Please know that if you don't hear from me in the weeks (and months?) after the birth, I'll be thinking of you!" Now you're officially off the hook.

- Invest in a nice reclining outdoor lounge chair if you'll be delivering in the summer or fall months, so you can nurse outside and enjoy some fresh air in those first few claustrophobic weeks.

- Get yourself a cute pedicure. It will be relaxing now, and later you can look at your cute little toes while you're in those stirrups!

- Nap, nap, nap.

- Buy yourself a top-of-the-line stroller, one that beckons you outdoors every single day. That way, you can plop the baby into the bucket seat and take off for the coffee shop—there's no sense in staying shut up in the house.

- Consider hiring a doula! She'll come to your house before the birth and get you prepared, sit by your side and soothe you throughout the birth, and then care for you and the baby once she's born. Doulas are like walking, talking instruments of nurture.

You *are* just the kind of parent your child is going to love having. In the next chapter, we'll learn all about what you can do over the first 2 years to set your baby on his or her way toward a long, happy, healthy life. You can do that without ever sacrificing your own happiness—and be a happy, healthy parent for years to come!

Chapter Eleven

Get It Right from the Start

You've gone through the all-consuming process of pregnancy and childbirth. And now you're lying in your hospital bed with this tiny miracle in your arms.

Now what?

You've read about how these early years can have an impact on your baby's life for a long time. In the process of getting to know your little miracle, you may find the first few days, weeks, months, years of your child's life to be a time of great exploration and growth . . . as well as exhaustion and self-denial. You'll learn more than you ever wanted to know about bowel movements, spit-up, and cradle cap, a minor skin condition that makes your adorable baby's head look like it's covered with dandruff. But you'll also learn a tremendous amount about your own emotional depths—how much fear of the unknown you have inside you, and also how much love.

Parenting infants and toddlers is incredibly physical work—the lifting, the carrying, the rocking, the not sleeping. Yet all of these daily tasks of nurturing and the physical closeness that they bring are what communicate our love to our kids before they can understand any words. You feel a deep sense of protectiveness, and your mama or papa bear nature comes out in full force. That's why you may find it tremendously reassuring to know that taking just a few steps now can set your child on the path to lifelong health.

Fix It in 5
Set the Stage for a Lifetime of Health

1. Breastfeed your baby and feed the whole family healthy, organic foods.
2. Encourage your child to adopt a regular sleep pattern as soon as possible.
3. Don't smoke around the baby.
4. Put an infant to sleep on his or her back.
5. "Spoil" your child with extra cuddle time.

Everything from what your family eats to how they move to what they read may help your baby live a longer, healthier, happier life. And here's a huge bonus: Many of the things that are best for junior—calming touch, extra sleep, breastfeeding—have health benefits for Mom and Dad, too. Let's take a look at what happens from the first moment in your child's life—and how within the first 2 years you can build a foundation of health that will sustain him or her for many decades to come.

A 5-Minute Tour of Your Baby's First 2 Years

If you look at every species on earth, in general, the more intelligent it is, the longer its childhood is. As a highly intelligent species, humans require a few decades to fully mature and develop (if we ever actually get there). Our babies are born completely unable to take care of themselves. That's our job. A newborn has basically three tasks:

- Eat (and burp)
- Sleep
- Fill diaper

As a new parent, you will likely be amazed at how much of your time these activities take up, even though these busy bees are incapable of holding up their heads and have poor vision, jittery reflexes, and trouble communicating in anything other than a loud wail or a low whimper. But within 3 months, newborns start to develop the basic skills and personality that will evolve and develop throughout their lives.

Zero to 3 Months: The Worm Stage

A newborn baby requires constant feeding, roughly every 2 or 3 hours, as well as frequent diaper changes. Beyond that, the best thing you can do for your new baby is to hold and cuddle him or her: Babies thrive near the warmth and smell of their caregivers and with lots of loving interactions with the people around them. Each of these encounters teaches a baby about the world and will aid in his or her development.

Babies are born with a sucking reflex and are capable of breastfeeding moments after birth—a reflex that comes in handy because they can also be pacified by sucking on a finger or a pacifier between feedings. They've just spent 9 months soaking in amniotic fluid, so their skin is wrinkled and shriveled—all the better to complement their puffy eyes, swollen from childbirth. No matter: Your baby will be the most beautiful creature you've ever laid eyes upon. (And those wrinkles will start to smooth out and plump up very quickly. Soon you'll be seeing lots of other folds, instead.)

The soft hair, or lanugo, that covers most of a newborn's body will begin to shed within a few days (if it hasn't been shed in the womb already), and she will start to gain weight as she feeds. Dads, don't get too proud of the size of your son's genitalia just yet. His scrotum—swollen from his mother's hormones within the womb—will start to recede. And soon, in just a few weeks, the wrinkly, puffy newborn you met after childbirth will look very different.

Other milestones of these months include:

- Lifts and turns head when lying on back
- Balls hands into fists, flexes arms
- Closes hand to grip your finger (palmar hand grasp)
- Flexes toes and forefeet (plantar grasp)
- Brings hands to eyes and mouth
- Follows an object moved in an arc about 6 inches above his face to the midline (right between his eyes, as he looks straight ahead)
- May turn head toward a familiar sound or voice
- Responds to noises with startling, crying, or quieting

3 to 6 Months: The Mirror Stage

At 3 months, your baby will develop the ability to smile at you, and will also become more playful and interactive. At this stage, babies can usually lift their heads, kick their legs, and open and shut their hands. They also may be able to grab or shake toys. Their vision starts to develop and they can watch faces or follow moving objects, and may recognize your face or voice and smile in response. The little gurgling noises they make may soon turn into babbling or even imitations of sounds. By this time, if you haven't already taken the dive, prepare to fall totally, completely in love.

Other milestones of these months include:

- Raises head 45 degrees during "tummy time"
- Uses arms to raise into a baby pushup (he'll be pumping iron in no time)
- Pushes feet down when stood on a flat surface
- Has increased control of eyes and ability to track objects
- Is deeply engaged with watching faces
- Smiles at the sound of Mom's and/or Dad's voice
- Begins to make noises intentionally
- Neck muscles strengthen, allowing her to eventually sit without support (at 5 to 6 months of age)
- Rolls from stomach to back
- May roll from back to stomach and grab for objects

7 to 9 Months: The Investigator Stage

Babies at this stage become very playful and interested in the world around them. Playing games like peekaboo or sitting together and reading colorful books will become endlessly fascinating. They should also begin to recognize and respond to their names, and may babble something in return. They begin to move more as they learn to roll, sit, reach for objects, and grab and shake objects. While previously your baby was probably happy with anyone who was willing to give him or her attention and cuddles, at this stage, he or she may develop stranger anxiety and prefer Mom or Dad to anyone else. Up until now, babies are probably content with milk, but as their teeth develop and their tastes mature, you can start to introduce soft foods to supplement the milk.

Other milestones of these months include:

- Crawling! (Now you're in for it . . .)
- Sits and plays for many minutes at a time
- Sits from a standing position
- May pull him- or herself up on furniture in order to stand
- Looks for dropped objects
- Responds to name
- Plays peekaboo
- Babbles

10 to 12 months: The Mover and Shaker Stage

By 12 months, though crawling like a champ, a baby becomes very attached to his parents. You may find your 12-month-old becoming very clingy and resistant to being left at day care or with a babysitter. But he is also starting to become independent—he can usually begin to feed himself finger foods, learn to walk and stand up, and speak basic words. At this point, your baby's weight has likely tripled from her birth weight, and she will continue to grow about ¼ to ½ inch each month.

Other milestones of these months include:

- Works to get toys that are out of reach
- Is crawling like a demon!
- Gets mad if toys are taken away
- Couch surfs (watch out for the remote)
- May say "mama" and "dada"—at first to anyone, but later specifically to Mom and Dad
- Starts to balance when standing alone
- May take first steps

12 to 18 Months: The Transitional Phase

At this stage, your baby is fast becoming a little person. By this point, he's likely to have tripled his birth weight and is now 150 percent taller than when he was born. He can stand up, walk with help (and soon will by himself), and has a strong pincer grasp that allows him to easily pick up the peas from his plate. He's struggling a bit with separation anxiety, but at the same time, he's starting to feel like his own man. He enjoys getting away for brief stretches to explore new settings and meet new friends—but he's always thrilled to come back to you.

Other milestones of these months include:

- No longer has a fontanelle (that soft spot on her head)
- Drinks from a cup (with help)
- Points to objects with her index finger
- Runs or crawls after fast-moving objects
- Picks up finger food more easily
- Tries to build small towers out of two or more blocks
- Responds to his name
- Can say "mama," "papa," and at least one or two other words
- Understands simple commands
- Tries to imitate animal sounds (*quack! ruff! moo!*)
- Looks for objects that are hidden, knowing they still exist (object constancy)
- Waves bye-bye
- Has a favorite "blankie" or toy

18 to 24 Months: The "Getting Into Everything" Stage

At this point, your little guy is probably ready to *go*. He does not understand why anything stands in his way. He can probably climb, walk, even run (although not very well; they aren't called toddlers for nothing). He falls a lot, but bounces right back, ready for more. He's starting to grow a little less slowly, and his appetite starts to slow down. (Don't worry, it's totally natural—*never* force a child to eat more than he's hungry for.) He's eager to learn to be a big kid, and he pretends constantly, maybe by imitating scribbling, reading books, using the potty (though he might not be ready to be potty trained for several months, if not years).

Other milestones of these months include:

- Walks up stairs while holding on with one hand
- Can use a spoon to feed himself
- Drinks through a straw
- Opens up cabinets and drawers (childproofing, anyone?)
- Climbs up onto chairs and up stairs by herself
- Identifies at least one body part
- Cuddles and shows affection
- Intently listens to rhymes
- Tries to hum and sing
- Will comfort a parent or friend who seems sad or distressed

24 to 36 months: The Independent Traveler Stage

When your child turns 2, her rate of growth slows down and her babylike appearance begins to change in this toddler stage as she becomes more active. Two-year-olds are traditionally called toddlers because they usually learn to walk and run independently and are curious about exploring the world. They typically like to climb, kick, throw, read books, talk and sing, and play with other children. Their vocabulary will include 200 to 300 words, and they begin to speak in simple sentences. While most 2-year-olds are learning to become independent, they often struggle with their limitations—giving rise to what is often called the terrible twos, which involves troubles with discipline and sharing and a tendency to see the world only from their own perspective. Adults have some of the same issues, don't they?

Other milestones of this year include:

- Walks alone
- Begins to run
- Kicks a ball
- Climbs on and off furniture unassisted
- Likes to pour things out of containers
- Builds block towers with four or more blocks
- Stands on tiptoe
- Becomes increasingly independent

5-Minute Fixes
for Your Little One's Lifetime of Great Health

We find it amazing—and inspiring—how absolutely obsessed new parents can become with giving their children the best possible start in life. It's in that spirit that we offer you these key fixes. Many take more than 5 minutes, and some require far less. But all have the potential to have tremendous, lifelong impacts on your children—and perhaps change the trajectory of your entire family tree!

Breast is best—for now and later. We know you've heard this, but we have to reiterate: There is no doubt that breastfeeding is absolutely the way that nature intended for us to feed our children. Breast milk actually develops babies' immune systems, giving them the antibodies necessary to fight infections. Breastfeeding may help protect babies against everything from stomach viruses, ear infections, and allergies to type 1 diabetes, sudden infant death syndrome (SIDS), celiac disease, colitis, and even childhood leukemias.

In fact, one review and meta-analysis of epidemiological studies analyzed the histories of 69,000 children, and when researchers controlled for all other health factors, they found that

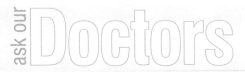
Is there any way to predict how tall
my toddler will be when he grows up?

Dr. Jim says . . .

Amazingly enough, we have a couple of ways to do this! One way is to ballpark it by simply doubling your child's height when he turns 2. Or, if your baby is still a little guy (or girl), you can use this handy calculation:

FOR BOYS

1. Take each parent's height in inches and add them together.
2. Divide that number by 2.
3. Add 2.5 inches to that number.
4. This number is the mid-parental height for boys.
5. This number plus or minus 4 inches is the height range you can reasonably expect your son to reach.

FOR GIRLS

1. Take each parent's height in inches and add them together.
2. Divide that number by 2.
3. Subtract 2.5 inches from that number.
4. This number is the mid-parental height for girls.
5. This number plus or minus 4 inches is the height range you can reasonably expect your daughter to reach.

Remember that these predictions are by no means guaranteed. Lots of factors determine the pattern and extent of your child's growth, including overall health and adequate nutrition and sleep. But these guidelines can help you predict your child's height based on our best guess of his genetic raw material: his parents!

breastfeeding lowered children's chances of becoming obese by almost 25 percent. The researchers also found that the longer a child breastfed, the lower his or her chances were of developing obesity in later childhood.

These effects are believed to carry over into adulthood. A World Health Organization study summarized the long-term effects and found that breastfed babies enjoyed improved cognitive development. And breastfeeding may also be associated with lower blood pressure and cholesterol levels in later years. The American Academy of Pediatrics recommends exclusive breastfeeding for the first 6 months, and then as long thereafter as mom and baby would prefer. Consider this the parenting gift that keeps on giving. **Time spent:** 10 to 15 minutes a feeding. **Time saved:** hours of sterilizing bottles, measuring formula, warming up mixed formula, earning extra money to buy formula . . .

Do it for yourself! For all of those selfless moms out there, we have a little secret to share: Breastfeeding is not just the best gift you can give your baby—it's good for you, too! In a study of almost 90,000 women who'd given birth, the results showed that, compared with women who had never breastfed, women who had breastfed for a lifetime total of 2 years or longer—even if it was with multiple babies!—had a 37 percent lower risk of coronary heart disease. Another study using the same group of women found that for each additional year the average woman breastfed, she had a 15 percent lower chance of developing type 2 diabetes. Australian researchers did their own study on 53,000 women and found that women who breastfed were 50 percent less likely to have type 2 diabetes than those who didn't. These scientists believe something happens during the breastfeeding process that may change the way you process glucose and insulin, offering protective effects that last long after you stop breastfeeding.

And speaking of weight: Breastfeeding burns an additional 500 calories a day, which may help you shed your postbaby pounds in the months after birth. Each time you nurse, your body will be bathed in a surge of oxytocin, the hormone related to milk release that also makes you feel loving, connected, and calm. (Talk about Mommy's Little Helper!) **Time spent:** 10 to

15 minutes a feeding, during which time you can talk on the phone, watch TV, read, or just stare lovingly at your gorgeous baby!

Be the poop police. Your pediatrician may ask you to track how many times your baby eats and poops during the day. You should certainly keep an eye on these things, but you don't need to be obsessive about it. Some breastfed babies will not have a bowel movement every day because their nutrition is so perfectly matched to their needs that there is less waste. That said, keep an eye out for signs that your baby may have constipation, a common issue in newborns.

The best stool is nice and mushy (perhaps "nice" and "mushy" and "stool" don't really seem to belong together, but you'll understand what we mean). Switching between breast milk and formula can cause constipation. So if you see any signs that your baby's belly is hurting or he's straining to pass a firm stool less than once a day; seems to have pain when passing a stool; or the poop is dry, hard, or pebble-shaped, be sure that you are drinking enough fluids. Breast-feeding moms should have a full, large glass of water every time they nurse, and steer clear of caffeinated beverages, which can be diuretics for you—and speed for your baby.

If after a day or so of constipation your baby still seems uncomfortable, check with your doctor—she may recommend that you give the baby a bit of water or extra meals, which will increase the fluid in the colon and stool. Give his belly a rub, let him relax in a warm bath, and "bicycle" his legs to help him work out any other intestinal trouble. **Time spent:** 1 minute to note his poops each time you change the diaper

Cuddle that bug—all day long. Once you've done your feeding and diapering, the last routine task of baby care is one of the best: cuddling. Touch is an essential ingredient in any baby's daily needs. While modern parents have thousands of baby furniture options—swings, bucket seats, bouncy chairs, oh my!—the best seat in the house is still your arms.

When babies are carried close to their parents' bodies in slings or other baby carriers for just 3 hours a day, it's been found that they cry 43 percent less total—54 percent less during the evening "witching hours." Studies have shown that "kangaroo care"—holding your

Doctors

Is the family bed okay—or even safe—for kids?

Dr. Jim says . . .

Co-sleeping—sharing your bed with your baby, toddler, or older kid—is a hot topic among parents, pediatricians, and consumer-safety groups. Proponents say sleeping with your baby can help her fall asleep faster, promote easy breastfeeding at night, make you bond more closely with your child, and—no small matter—maybe help a tired parent get more shut-eye.

Keeping your baby close is a natural instinct—and in fact, sleeping in the same room could, according to the *American Academy of Pediatrics,* even reduce her risk for SIDS. But on the other side of the issue are serious concerns about infant death caused by parents rolling over in their sleep or by the baby becoming trapped and even suffocating on a waterbed mattress or in soft bedding. That's why the Consumer Product Safety Commission recommends never sleeping with a baby or child under the age of 2.

newborn baby skin-to-skin between your breasts under your clothing—has even more dramatic results, intensifying your attachment to your baby, helping to prevent postpartum depression, and helping to establish successful, long-lasting breastfeeding. One study found that playing lullabies during 60 minutes of kangaroo care helped preemies cry less and sleep more deeply, and helped their moms feel less anxious. Overall, kangaroo care enhances every aspect of your relationship with your baby, including her physical and mental development, and sets her up for a longer, happier, healthier life. Not bad for a bit of snuggling, huh? **Time spent:** as much as possible!

Moms feed and love, dads play and love. Parents reap significant benefits from these interactions, as well. In one study of 160 families, researchers found that the more the moms

Experts acknowledge that many parents will decide to sleep with a baby or young child nearby or in the same bed despite the concerns. For the safest slumber, they recommend these strategies:

Try room sharing instead of bed sharing. Put your baby's bed beside yours. You could use a regular bassinet, a crib, or a co-sleeper bassinet with a removable side.

Practice safer co-sleeping. If you do plan to share a bed, baby-proof it first. Be sure there are no spaces between the mattress and the wall or nearby furniture, or at the headboard or footboard, where the baby's head could become trapped. Remove soft bedding and pillows from the bed, as well as curtains and cords from nearby windows. Put a tight-fitting sheet on the bed. Be sure your pajamas and your baby's don't have any strings or ties. Make sure your baby is on her back with her head uncovered. Don't let the baby become overheated—and don't put her to sleep in an adult bed by herself.

Always skip co-sleeping if: You smoke (smoking in her presence raises the risk for SIDS), are extremely overweight, or may not be able to wake up quickly due to alcohol consumption, medication use, or sleep apnea. Skip it if you sleep on a waterbed or a soft, squishy mattress, and if you are drowsing on a couch. And never let a babysitter, siblings, or other adults sleep with the baby.

touched their babies affectionately and spoke with them in singsongy "motherese," the higher their blood levels of oxytocin, the aforementioned cuddle hormone that's known to lower blood pressure, decrease levels of stress hormones and depression, and increase feelings of connection and contentment. Dads got the same benefit from playing with their babies in a physical way—moving their arms and legs around, pretending to make them dance, and other crazy things new dads like to do. These interactions are also fantastic for a baby's brain because they stimulate new connections and help her feel loved and excited to learn. **Time spent:** as much as possible!

Create a "feeding station" in each room. One of the hardest things about parenting a newborn can be the sense of isolation—sometimes bordering on captivity—that you can feel when you're nursing every 2 hours. Rather than having one place to feed the baby, keep a stash of supplies in each room. You'll need: A large glass for water, a pillow or two (for correct posture), a few receiving blankets or spit pads, a footstool, and a television remote/telephone/copy of *People* magazine nearby. **Time spent:** about 5 minutes a day replenishing your station supplies will give you maximum enjoyment and convenience throughout the day

Wipe those gums after each feeding. Most people don't think about their babies' oral health until they see that first shiny tooth. But preventing tooth decay starts within the first few days of your child's life. After each feeding, wet a small piece of gauze or a baby washcloth and rub it gently over your baby's gums to prevent any bacteria or plaque from forming. Once the first tooth comes in, put a tiny dab of nonfluoride toothpaste on the gauze before you wipe, and encourage your baby to spit after you're done. Your child's first dentist visit should occur between age 3 and 4, unless there is a specific dental or oral problem.

Above all, please don't allow your baby to fall asleep at the breast or with a bottle. Instead, try to lay him down in his crib awake. This will not only give you a chance to clean out his mouth, he'll also learn to soothe himself to sleep, which will lead to better sleep habits and prevent a boob-to-sleep addiction! **Time spent:** 30 seconds after each feeding

Stick with the bottle or boob for at least 6 months. We get a lot of questions from parents about how to keep their kids from developing food allergies, and we're going to be honest—we think some of the books out there are wrong. We need to give those little baby immune systems time to develop before we start challenging them with a lot of different foods. A kid's guts—intestines—act as a filter that matures over time. When they're really young, that filter is open and everything just leaks through into the body, absorbing not only the good stuff, but also some potential allergens. As the gut matures, it becomes "smarter," and the immune system learns to recognize potential allergens and block them from being absorbed. But when kids get certain foods too early—especially the ones that most commonly cause allergies, like milk, nuts, and soy—they can develop allergies. And those last for a long, long time.

Doctors

My kid is a puker—it seems like he's always spitting up. How do I know when it's time to take him to the doctor?

Dr. Jim says . . .

There's a big difference between "spitting up" and puking—and believe me, when puking happens, you know the difference. Babies spit up right after they eat if they're not burped adequately—burping settles their stomachs and makes room for milk. Some babies will have the infant version of acid reflux, which causes them to spit up more often. But you can help your baby by laying him on his belly across your knees and rubbing his back, or by moving his legs in a bicycling motion—both of these actions may help settle his stomach. Of course, see your pediatrician if your baby seems to be in pain.

True puking (vomiting) is distinguished by volume and by force—puke really flies out, where as spit-up kind of dribbles. Vomiting can be caused by a bacterial or viral infection, a systemic illness, or a toxin.

The vomiting itself isn't a big deal; it's the dehydration that results that's the problem. I tell my patients they can start to worry when their child:

- Has not peed in several hours (6 to 8 hours for younger kids and 10 to 12 hours for older kids)
- Is irritable or lethargic
- Has skin "tenting," which means that if you pinch the skin on the back of her hand, it does not retract when you let go
- Has a sunken-in soft spot on his or her head
- Has lost more than 10 percent of his or her body weight

If your child is getting sick, it's important to start giving electrolyte drinks, juices, frozen juice pops, or broth right away to keep him hydrated and prevent him from getting lethargic. But if he does seem lethargic, take him to the ER for intravenous fluids because he may not be taking in enough fluids orally to keep up with what he's losing by vomiting.

Keep it simple! Stick exclusively to the breast or the bottle for the first 6 months. Enjoy those efficient feeds while you can—bottle- and breastfeeding are way faster than chopping, scooping, wiping chins, cleaning up, hosing down. After 6 months, you can add in one food at a time. Here's a list from the Web site that Dr. Jim shares with his dad, Dr. Bill Sears. Favorite First Foods:

- rice cereal
- peaches
- barley cereal
- applesauce
- bananas
- carrots
- pears
- squash
- avocados
- sweet potatoes

(Check out a fuller description of "Starting Solid Foods," at www.askdrsears.com/html/3/T032000.asp.) **Time spent:** 10 to 15 minutes per feeding versus 30 minutes or more

Open that jar. When it's time to transition to solid foods, very well-intentioned parents who are trying to do everything possible for their babies ask us if it's really okay to use jarred food. Well, not only is it okay, it can be preferable. Some vegetables are naturally high in nitrates, which, according to researchers at Clemson University in South Carolina, can be dangerous for a baby under 6 months old. In the body, those nitrates change into nitrites, which can bind with iron in the blood and make breathing difficult. Use caution when serving your baby beets, broccoli, cabbage, carrots, celery, collard greens, lettuce, spinach, or turnips by reaching for organic jarred versions (they're always nitrate-free). Wait until your baby is a year or older before you serve him the homemade versions of these vegetables. Don't believe organic is worth

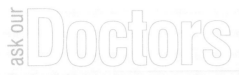

My husband "cleans" off our baby's pacifier—in his own mouth! Is this okay?

Dr. Jim says . . .

Actually, no. Here's the thing: Your baby is born without any of the bacteria that cause cavities. Where does he get those germs from? You! You pass it along in your saliva—by sharing spoons and testing foods before you give it to him, and even by blowing on hot food. So when your husband "cleans" the pacifier, he's essentially loading it up with extra germs. Urge your husband to run the pacifier under warm water instead. To further guard against germ transfer, make sure you and your husband brush your teeth with fluoride toothpaste after each meal, and if you have bleeding gums or cavities, see your dentist ASAP.

the extra cost? Try both kinds yourself—you'll see that the organic varieties taste more like the real thing, and they don't have all of those extra pesticides or, in the case of meat, hormones. You can even supplement your jarred organic baby foods with foods that are naturally mushy—avocados (a great source of omega-3 fatty acids), bananas, applesauce, and yogurt.

Time spent: 15 seconds to twist off that cap

Please get your baby vaccinated. We know this is a tremendously hot-button issue, and we can certainly appreciate everyone's concern. We even share differences of opinion among the four of us. But you should know that the CDC considers vaccinations to be one of the 10 greatest public health advances of the 20th century.

Take, for example, the chicken pox vaccine. Some parents consider it an optional vaccine, and some even expose their children to the virus intentionally by having them attend "chicken pox parties" so they'll get their immunity "the natural way."

But these parents aren't aware that chicken pox is a potentially deadly disease. Most people develop sores on the skin and mouth, but sometimes the virus infects the lungs, brain, heart, or joints. These complications happen more often in newborns, adults, and people with immune system problems than in otherwise healthy children. Chicken pox is fatal in up to 15 percent of people who have an impaired immune system.

Now consider a new study published in *The Pediatric Infectious Disease Journal*. Before the introduction of the vaccine in 1995, about 90 percent of children caught chicken pox by age 15. Since the vaccine was introduced in 1995, the rate of chicken pox-related office visits among children zero to 4 years old has decreased by *98 percent*.

If you are worried about your baby receiving too many vaccines at once, consider reading books on this topic, which may help you articulate some of your concerns to your doctor.

But once you've shared them, listen to what he or she has to say, listen to your gut, make a decision, and then don't second-guess yourself. Except in very rare cases, the risk-benefit ratio of most vaccines is very clear: Vaccines save lives. **Time spent:** 5 minutes at each pediatrician visit to share concerns and ask questions

Look for a preschool or day care near green space. When you're calling to make appointments to look at child care facilities, ask right away, "Are you near a highway?" A recent study in the journal *Environmental Health Perspectives* suggests that kids who attend schools near high-traffic areas have a 45 percent increased risk of asthma. Asthma is the most common chronic childhood illness in developed countries. But asthma is not the only childhood illness caused by environmental pollutants—and not the only one whose incidence could be decreased with better air quality. A recent study from researchers at UCLA and Brigham and Women's Hospital in Boston reviewed National Health Interview Survey data for more than 120,000 children and found that improvements in air quality that have occurred since the Clean Air Act was passed in 1970 have greatly reduced the number of chronic ear infections.

Make it a priority to find a day care provider or center that has a garden or a lawn. This green space will keep your child's respiratory system healthy, and schools placed in nature have

My second daughter was born 4 weeks ago
and has not gained any weight since she was
discharged from the hospital. I'm breastfeeding
her. Could my breast milk be deficient?

Dr. Jim says . . .

Most newborns will lose a few ounces right after birth, but it is important that they regain the lost weight within a week or, at the longest, 2 weeks.

If your baby is already 4 weeks old and hasn't regained the weight she lost right after birth, I'd be concerned about that. First off, you need to make sure your doctor is checking the baby. Make sure the baby looks okay, and then your doctor and maybe a lactation consultant can check your milk supply by pumping your breasts or weighing the baby before and after feeding to see if you're making enough milk. If you aren't, you may want to supplement with a little formula, just to get the baby back up to birth weight, because it's really important that she does that to stay healthy.

also been shown to reduce behavioral problems among the children. If you can't find one with a yard, try to find one as far removed from major roads and highways as possible—even a school tucked away on the second floor of a building at an office park is preferable to a small center located along a busy road. **Time spent:** 2 minutes per screening phone call

Put the paddle away. The National Poll on Children's Health from the University of Michigan C.S. Mott Children's Hospital found that the vast majority of parents— 88 percent—used explanation or reason to help set their misbehaving kids straight and 62 percent put their kids in a time-out. But while many parents avoid spanking as a disciplinary technique, a swat on the butt still remains a go-to technique for 30 percent of today's parents of toddlers and preschoolers. If you're inclined to think, "Hey, it worked for my parents," just remember that we know a lot more about the developing mind now than we did 30 or 40 years ago. Research shows that kids who are spanked are more likely to grow up to be aggressive—they may get the message that when you disagree with someone, the way to solve it is with physical violence. Worse still, it may teach our youngsters that hitting *is* love—and they'll unconsciously choose partners who will give them just that kind of "love."

Please consider using alternative means of disciplining your child. Start by increasing

Symptoms: Runny and/or stuffy nose; sneezing; attempts at throat clearing; itchy, watery red eyes. Symptoms last for more than a week or two, and may return at the same time each year.
What it could mean: Allergy
What to do: See your pediatrician or an allergist for an evaluation.

Symptoms: Coughing, wheezing, chest tightness, difficulty breathing; it may happen more at night or when your child is physically active
What it could mean: Asthma
What to do: See your pediatrician for an evaluation.

Symptoms: Runny nose and complaints of ear pain or tugging at the ears; may be accompanied by a fever
What it could mean: Ear infection
What to do: Call your pediatrician.

Symptoms: Severe sore throat, swollen glands, a fever of 101°F or higher, possibly with a stomachache or rash on the belly
What it could mean: Strep throat or another throat infection
What to do: Call your pediatrician.

Symptoms: Runny nose with thick or colored discharge, headache, sometimes with fever
What it could mean: Sinus infection
What to do: Call your pediatrician.

the positive encounters you have with your kids—experts say the best parenting ratio is five or six positive experiences to every negative experience. Be a model of kindness, starting with how you treat them. Encourage them to be honest and to play fair, and acknowledge it when they work hard to accomplish something. Reinforcing good behavior instead of punishing bad will be more effective in the long run. **Time spent:** varies; it takes more time to talk with your child than to spank, but the dividends will pay off for his entire life

Leave "grazing" to the cows. Thirty years ago, only three out of four kids would snack

Doctors

I'm so nervous about autism. My daughter is
2 and I don't think her language abilities are developing very quickly. How can I tell if she's autistic?

Dr. Jim says . . .

Most kids start talking at about 12 months or so. By 18 months, we like to see kids have a pretty good vocabulary, at least 10 words and sometimes up to maybe 50 words. But they don't need to be saying them all correctly; if you can understand half of what they say, that's okay. If your daughter is 2 now, she should have a huge vocabulary, but instead of "doggie" she'll likely be saying "oggie." At age 2, she should be saying two-word phrases and short sentences. If she's not doing this, or if she's showing some regression—like going from being able to stand and trying to take steps to not being able to sit unsupported—then it's time to see the doctor. You might get her hearing tested as well.

Autism is a complicated developmental disorder called a spectrum disorder because the symptoms and the severity of the condition can vary greatly. Most commonly, autism affects a person's ability to correctly process emotions, language, and sensations. About 1 in every 110 kids in America will be diagnosed with autism. No one is certain what causes the disorder, and the subject is being hotly debated across the country. Currently, there is no known cure.

Autism is usually diagnosed between the ages of 3 and 6 years old, but symptoms usually surface much earlier. That's why it's so important for parents to know what milestones to watch for in their infant or toddler. Keep an eye out for these warning signs:

- Makes little or no eye contact
- Shows a lack of social engagement
- Has changes in social interaction

between meals, but now, it's practically mandatory—98 percent of kids do it every day. The concept of mini-meals caught on big time in the '90s, but a recent study may reveal a dark side of this eating pattern. A study in the journal *Health Affairs* found that kids who eat snacks an average of three times a day are eating junk like chips, candy, and other nutrition-

- Appears to be in his or her own world
- Has no interest in playing with other children
- Shows no attachment to parents
- Is unaware of the environment or other people
- Has a speech delay or shows changes in verbal skills, meaning that he or she either doesn't learn to talk or has regressed and stopped talking
- Exhibits repetitive behaviors like hand flapping, staring at ceiling fans, spinning or rocking, or lining up toy cars or other objects
- Doesn't "pretend" play
- Can't point with the index finger
- Regresses or loses skills at any time

For a complete list of autism warning signs from the Centers for Disease Control and Prevention, go to www.cdc.gov/ncbddd/autism/signs.html.

Your child should begin to make eye contact with you as an infant and respond to you with a smile by about 3 months of age. If at 5 months old your child is not smiling, or if your 6- to 9-month-old dislikes playing peekaboo, talk to your pediatrician. Not every child is talking by the 1st birthday, but a typical 12-month-old says at least "mama" and "dada" and can point with the index finger. If your child seems unresponsive or at any time loses a skill that's been learned, that's a warning sign. Repetitive behaviors, spinning, or rocking may also indicate autism. If your child is exhibiting any of these, seek the advice of your doctor.

Brains can heal with aggressive early intervention. Research at the University of Washington has shown that an autistic child's IQ, language ability, and social-interaction skills can be improved if the disorder is detected early. Treatments for autism, some of which can begin as early as 18 months of age, are incredibly diverse, ranging from applied behavior analysis to sessions in a hyperbaric chamber to working with animals. Experts have seen amazing results. If you're concerned, definitely speak up *now*.

ally bankrupt stuff—and those calories add up to more than a quarter of their daily intake. In the past 30 years, the average daily diet has stretched to accommodate 168 extra calories from snacking. (Toddlers, preschoolers, and kindergartners were the worst offenders, adding 182 snack calories per day.)

Let's try to reverse this trend of three meals and three snacks a day and get it back to one snack a day for school-age kids, two for kids 5 and younger. Focus on fruits, vegetables, and lean protein: Cut-up apples, low-fat cheese sticks, yogurt, fruit smoothies (throw some spinach in there!), hummus, and baby carrots are good choices. **Time spent:** about 5 minutes a day planning and preparing a healthy, satisfying snack (versus just opening a bag or a box)

Have family reading time for 5 minutes a day. One fascinating study that analyzed historical information from the US Census found that the three factors that determined the longevity of 85-year-old African Americans were growing up on a farm, having literate parents, and living in a two-adult household. While many of us can no longer give our children the farm experience, we can certainly give them the gifts of a stable relationship and a love of learning. Combine these two critical facets into one with family reading time every day—gather up your child's favorite books and seat him between you and your spouse on the couch. Take turns reading pages to your child as he basks in the warmth of parental love. That intense, focused attention is like Miracle-Gro for his soul. **Time spent:** 5 minutes a day for memories (and benefits) that will last a lifetime

Hold your temper with your spouse. A Swedish study looked at the histories of members of the Swedish population who were 77 or older in the years 1992 and 2002. They found that when the subjects' childhood homes had been filled with conflict, they had lower levels of cognition later in life. No matter what happened to those kids in those later years—if they succeeded in school, got good jobs, earned more money than their parents—those effects from the conflict remained. Before you stumble thoughtlessly into a fight with your spouse about something like the laundry or the bills, think about how these frequent small arguments now might affect your son or daughter down the road. If you feel yourself wanting to snap back, just take a deep breath and count to 10. Visualize that every second you resist yelling back will add an extra point to your child's IQ—because, who knows? It just might. **Time spent:** 30 deep-breathing-filled seconds

Trash those Twinkies. It's a proven fact: Overweight kids become overweight adults. But you can help set a good foundation for your children before they head off to school and face all the sugar-filled temptations that fill kids' lives every day.

First, don't ignore chubby baby syndrome. Our culture coos over those baby rolls, but they really are unhealthy. A recent study in the *Journal of Pediatrics* found that babies with those adorable Michelin Man levels of chub were more than twice as likely as lean babies to have low scores on motor skill development tests.

But as parents, we can live in a state of denial. More than 70 percent of parents believe their kids are getting enough exercise—when they're not. Among kids who are overweight, *83 percent* will remain overweight as adults. And if we're carrying a few extra pounds as well, we might as well be force-feeding them junk food. They're almost destined to get fat: Children of obese parents are *13 times more likely* to become obese than children of normal-weight parents.

But enough hand-wringing! You have a great opportunity to stop that trajectory now. Be a great example for your kids: Eat well, exercise, lose excess weight. Turn off the television. Don't have junk food in the house. Snack on fruits, vegetables, nuts, and low-fat dairy products. Make sure everyone gets enough shut-eye.

But keep your eyes open. Don't be complacent. Now is the time to make that change. **Time spent:** 15 minutes to go through your cabinets and toss the junk food; 15 minutes to plan the week's meals and write up a grocery list

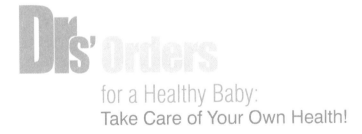

Drs' Orders for a Healthy Baby: Take Care of Your Own Health!

This "Doctors' Orders" might surprise you—how could taking care of yourself be the most important thing you can do for your baby? Simple: You are your baby's world. Your baby learns everything about the world from the way you live. If you are calm, peaceful, and loving, she will absorb that energy and learn that the world is calm, peaceful, and loving. If you spend time taking care of your body, sleeping enough, laughing with friends—she will learn to value these things as well. You will have more energy, more enthusiasm, more of everything to give to her—but you must first give it to yourself.

The job of being a parent is never ending, so you can't just wait until the baby grows up before you take care of yourself again. If you do that, you'll never recover! Just as a baby needs to be diapered, fed, and rocked every single day, your body and soul need to be nurtured as well.

Starting to do this—eating well, exercising, sleeping at least 7 hours a night (or day!), getting plenty of downtime with your spouse and friends—as early as possible in your baby's life means that your child will have the best example from the very first moment he becomes aware. His memories, looking back, will be of a happy mother or father who made health a priority. We live what we know—if your child knows only health, he will grow up with an intuitive ability to give his body what it needs to thrive.

And don't forget—honoring your emotional and intellectual needs is important as well. Don't move through life saying, "When the kids get older, I can't wait to . . ." Don't wait. Whatever it is, do it now. When you live your dreams, your kids will benefit more than you can possibly imagine. And in so doing, you'll be kicking off the first generation of a positive, healthy evolution that may reach your grandchildren, your great-grandchildren, and so on, through many generations of exceptional health. With your first 5-minute health fix today, you could change the health patterns, the degree of happiness, even the longevity of generations of your genetic offspring. And that's the very definition of creating time.

I've heard that nonorganic blueberries have a lot of pesticides—but I can't afford organic. But I've also heard that pesticides are linked to ADHD and other health problems, and I don't want to poison my kids. What should I do: buy the nonorganic or steer clear entirely?

There is more and more evidence to suggest potential harms of exposure to pesticide residues on food, although the evidence is still less than definitive. However, intuition suggests that such exposures certainly can't be a good thing!

That said, the scientific literature linking higher intake of fruits and vegetables to better health outcomes is vast, consistent, and definitive. What tends to go unsaid is this: those studies just about never distinguish organic from conventionally grown produce. In other words, more plant foods are good for us even despite any harms of pesticide residues.

So if you can find and afford organic blueberries, by all means go for it—they are likely better for you, and certainly better for the planet. But if you can't find, or afford, organic berries, eat berries anyway, and just rinse them well in cold water. Rinsing will remove nearly all pesticide, and the intrinsic benefits of eating blueberries will trump the potential harms of any trace left behind.

—*David Katz, MD, MPH, FACPM, FACP,* director,
Prevention Research Center at the Yale University School of Medicine

Test Taking Is Not Just for Kids

You've seen how the average person can do a tremendous amount for his or her health in just 5 minutes a day. But sometimes you need a bit more information to go on, more data about the state of your insides. Your doctor will advise you on what are the best tests for your age and health status, but here is a good look at many of the medical tests recommended at each phase of life.

Which Tests Do You Need?

Some tests are specific to your family and medical history; some are general tests that almost everyone gets. Here's a look at the basics, age by age.

SCREENING TESTS FOR NEWBORNS

- Screening tests for congenital disorders (screening guidelines vary from state to state, but most likely the screening tests will include phenylketonuria, congenital hypothyroidism, sickle-cell anemia, and a host of other inherited disorders)
- Hearing impairment
- Iron deficiency (complete blood count test)
- Lead poisoning (if a child lives in an old house with lead paint or a parent works with lead)
- Tuberculosis (if in contact with someone who has or may have tuberculosis)

SCREENING TESTS FOR CHILDREN (AGES 2 TO 12)

Note: Other than their usual hearing and vision tests, children aren't likely to need additional screening. However, in some cases the following screening tests are warranted.

- Obesity (body mass index)
- Diabetes (If a kid is overweight, has a family history of diabetes, and is in a high-risk ethnic group such as African Americans, he or she should be screened every 2 years for diabetes, starting at 10 years of age or at the onset of puberty if that occurs earlier. Screening involves glucose testing and sometimes a glucose tolerance test.)
- High cholesterol (if there is a family history of heart disease or high cholesterol or if the child is overweight)

- Lead poisoning (if living in an old house with lead paint or a parent works with lead)
- Tuberculosis (if in contact with someone who has or may have tuberculosis)

SCREENING TESTS FOR TEENS (AGES 13 TO 18)

- Obesity
- Cervical cancer (if a girl is sexually active, she will need a Pap test)
- Chlamydia and gonorrhea (if a girl is sexually active)
- Diabetes
- High cholesterol
- HIV (if at risk)
- Tuberculosis (if in contact with someone who has or may have tuberculosis)

SCREENING TESTS FOR YOUNG ADULTS (AGES 19 TO 29)

- Breast cancer (a health care professional will check the breasts for lumps)
- Cervical cancer (Pap test)
- Chlamydia and gonorrhea
- High cholesterol
- HIV
- Obesity
- Diabetes
- Tuberculosis (if in contact with someone who has or may have tuberculosis)

SCREENING TESTS FOR ADULTS (AGES 30 TO 49)

- Breast cancer (a health care professional will check the breasts for lumps)
- Cervical cancer (Pap test)
- High cholesterol
- Obesity
- HIV
- Thyroid dysfunction (most commonly, thyroid stimulating hormone blood test)

- Chlamydia and gonorrhea
- Colorectal cancer (if there is a family history you may need a colorectal cancer fecal occult blood test or colonoscopy)
- Diabetes
- Osteoporosis (bone density scan)
- Prostate cancer (if a family history or African American; could be a digital rectal exam or possibly a prostate-specific antigen [PSA] test)
- Tuberculosis (if in contact with someone who has or may have tuberculosis)

SCREENING TESTS FOR ADULTS (AGES 50 AND UP)

- Breast cancer (time for a mammogram!)
- Cervical cancer (probably needed less frequently than annually—or may even be stopped—if a history of normal Pap test results)
- Colorectal cancer (colonoscopy)
- High cholesterol
- HIV
- Obesity
- Osteoporosis (bone density scan)
- Thyroid dysfunction
- Chlamydia and gonorrhea
- Prostate cancer (digital rectal exam or PSA blood test)
- Tuberculosis (if in contact with someone who has or may have tuberculosis)

What Takes Place during a Routine Checkup?

Every checkup you have is an opportunity for your doctor to perform routine assessments.

In every checkup, your doctor should at least talk to you about:

- Blood pressure
- Height and weight

- Immunization status (the Centers for Disease Control and Prevention recommends particular vaccines based on age, occupation, health status, and other factors)
- Oral health
- Vision and hearing (as appropriate for your age)

Calculate Your BMI

One of the most versatile measures for healthy weight is the BMI, or body mass index, a ratio of your height and your weight. While the BMI is controversial (many experts prefer body composition instead, which measures precisely how much fat versus muscle you have in your body), it can provide a quick and easy snapshot of your risks of developing many common diseases.

Here's a formula you can use to figure out your BMI with pen and paper. If this looks too complicated—we think it does!—you can go to www.nhlbisupport.com/bmi and have a computer do it for you.

Step 1: Square your height (in inches). So if you are 65 inches high,

$$65 \times 65 = 4,225.$$

Step 2: Divide your weight (in pounds) by that number. So if you weigh 150 pounds,

$$150 \div 4225 = 0.0355029586.$$

Step 3: Multiply that number by 703. So in this case,

$$0.0355029586 \times 703 = 25. \text{ This is your BMI.}$$

WHAT DOES THE BMI NUMBER MEAN?
- Underweight = less than 18.5
- Normal weight = 18.5 to 24.9
- Overweight = 25 to 29.9
- Obesity = 30 or greater

Sharing Your Family History

Family history is one of the best sources of useful information for your doctor. Rather than trying to scour your memory bank in the few minutes you have when you're with your doctor, collect this information beforehand and you'll always have it at the ready.

Research and fill out this chart before heading to the doctor. This is just a sample; adjust the rows to match your biological family.

MY PERSONAL INFORMATION

Age: _____ years

Height: _____ inches

Weight: _____ pounds

BMI: _____ (see formula on opposite page to figure out your BMI)

	STILL LIVING?	HEART DISEASE (Y/N)	STROKE (Y/N)	DIABETES (Y/N)	COLON CANCER (Y/N)	BREAST CANCER (Y/N)	OVARIAN CANCER (Y/N)	ADDITIONAL DISEASES OR CONDITIONS
Self								
Child								
Father								
Mother								
Brother								
Sister								
Paternal grandfather								
Paternal grandmother								
Paternal aunt								
Paternal uncle								
Maternal grandfather								
Maternal grandmother								
Maternal aunt								

Chart Your Cholesterol

The lipid profile is one of the best-known blood tests, and knowing your targets can help you set goals with your primary care doctor or cardiologist. New research from doctors at Johns Hopkins University suggests that your hemoglobin A1c (HbA1c) level, which reflects the amount of sugar that has been in your blood over the past few months, is also a good indicator of the risk of future heart disease.

BLOOD VALUE	WHAT IS IT?	DANGER ZONE	AVERAGE TO BORDER-LINE RANGE	AVERAGE TO OPTIMAL RANGE
Total cholesterol	The sum of HDL, LDL, and VLDL (very-low-density-lipoprotein)	240 mg/dL or higher	200–239 mg/dL	Less than 200 mg/dL
High-density lipoprotein, or HDL ("good" cholesterol)	A fat that takes extra cholesterol in the bloodstream to the liver for disposal; high levels protect against cardiovascular disease	Less than 40 mg/dL for men; less than 50 mg/dL for women	40–50 mg/dL for men; 50–59 mg/dL for women	Higher than 50 mg/dL for men or 60 mg/dL for women—the higher the better
Low-density lipoprotein, or LDL ("bad" cholesterol)	A fat that is deposited in blood vessel walls; high levels contribute to hardening of the arteries	160 mg/dL or higher (190 mg/dL or higher is very high)	130–159 mg/dL	Less than 129 mg/dL (less than 100 mg/dL is best)
Triglyceride	A fat that circulates in blood, provides fuel for muscles; high levels linked with heart disease	200 mg/dL or higher (500 mg/DL or higher is very high)	150–199 mg/dL	Less than 150 mg/dL
HbA1c, or glycated hemoglobin	A measurement that indicates your blood sugar control over the previous few months; higher levels linked with heart disease	6.5% or higher	6–6.4%	5.9% or less (less than 5% is best)
Highly sensitive C-reactive protein, or hs-CRP	A measurement of proteins whose production increases with systemic inflammation; higher levels indicate a greater risk of adverse coronary events	3 milligrams per liter (mg/L) or higher	1–2.9 mg/L	Less than 1 mg/L

Blood Sugar and Insulin Response

With ever-increasing numbers of Americans developing insulin resistance and prediabetes, we'll see more and more testing of blood sugar in years to come. Familiarize yourself with these ranges to get a feel for where you stand on this continuum.

BLOOD VALUE	WHAT IS IT?	DANGER ZONE (DIABETIC)	AVERAGE TO BORDERLINE (PREDIABETIC) RANGE	OPTIMAL RANGE (NORMAL)
HbA1c, or glycated hemoglobin	A measurement that indicates your blood sugar control over the previous few months	6.5% or higher	6–6.4%	5.9% or less (less than 5% is best)
Fasting blood glucose	A measure of your blood sugar after an 8-hour fast	126 mg/dL (7.0 milli-moles per liter [mmol/L]) or more	100 to 125 mg/dL (5.6 to 6.9 mmol/L)	70 to 99 mg/dL (3.9 to 5.5 mmol/L)
Oral glucose tolerance test	A measurement of your body's reaction to a glucose drink after an 8-hour fast; blood is drawn every 30 to 60 minutes after you drink the solution; test can take up to 3 hours	More than 200 mg/dL (11.1 mmol/L or more)	140 to 200 mg/dL (7.8 to 11.0mmol/L)	Less than 140 mg/dL (7.7 mmol/L or less)

Oral Glucose Tolerence Test During Pregnancy

If the results of an oral glucose tolerance test meet or exceed two or more of the following values, gestational diabetes is diagnosed.

- Fasting (prior to taking the glucose): 95 mg/dL (5.3 mmol/L)
- 1 hour after taking the glucose: 180 mg/dL (10.0 mmol/L)
- 2 hours after taking the glucose: 155 mg/dL (8.6 mmol/L)
- 3 hours after taking the glucose: 140 mg/dL (7.8 mmol/L)

Complete Blood Count

As the name implies, this test gives a good idea of the health of your blood, which is important in diagnosing blood-related diseases ranging from anemia to leukemia.

Here are the various components of the test with the normal ranges listed.

- Red blood cell (RBC) count (varies with altitude):

  Males: 4.7 to 6.1 million cells per microliter (mcL)

  Females: 4.2 to 5.4 million cells/mcL
- White blood cell (WBC) count: 4,500 to 10,000 cells/mcL
- Hematocrit (the percentage of the blood that is RBCs; varies with altitude):

  Males: 40.7 to 50.3 percent

  Females: 36.1 to 44.3 percent
- Hemoglobin (a protein in RBCs that carries oxygen; varies with altitude):

  Males: 13.8 to 17.2 g/dL

  Females: 12.1 to 15.1 g/dL
- MCV (average red blood cell size): 80 to 95 femtoliters
- MCH (amount of hemoglobin in each RBC): 27 to 31 picograms per cell
- MCHC (the hemoglobin concentration in each RBC): 32 to 36 g/dL

Note: Normal value ranges may vary slightly among laboratories. Talk to your doctor about your specific test results.

HIGH RBC NUMBER COULD MEAN

- Dehydration (such as from severe diarrhea)
- Kidney disease

LOW RBC NUMBER COULD MEAN

- Anemia
- Leukemia
- Hemorrhage
- Multiple myeloma

LOW WBC NUMBER COULD MEAN

- Lupus
- Bone marrow disease
- Disease of the liver or spleen

HIGH WBC NUMBER COULD MEAN

- Infectious disease
- Arthritis or allergies
- Leukemia

Determine Your Flexibility

A study published in *American Journal of Physiology—Heart and Circulatory Physiology* described a novel way to test the flexibility of your arteries: Sit on the floor with your legs stretched out flat in front of you. If you are able to lean forward far enough to touch your toes, researchers found, your arteries are most likely flexible and less likely to have calcification and deposits.

As we get older, flexibility is also a good gauge of our risk of falls and other debilitating musculoskeletal injuries. Flexibility tests usually involve measurement devices such as the Acuflex, but you can use this modified test from the YMCA to test your flexibility at home.

1. Place the yardstick on the floor with the zero mark closest to you. Tape the yardstick in place at the 15-inch mark.

2. Ask a friend to help you keep your legs straight during the sit-and-reach test. However, it is important that he or she not interfere with your movement.

PROCEDURE

1. Warm up properly. Warmup activities include fast walking, jogging in place, or cycling on a stationary bicycle. Adding extra arm movements to these activities, like pumping your arms, will warm up your upper body.

2. Sit on the floor with the yardstick between your legs, your feet 10 to 12 inches apart, and the bottoms of your heels even with the tape at the 15-inch mark.

3. Place one hand over the other. The tips of your two middle fingers should be on top of one another.

4. Slowly stretch forward without bouncing or jerking, sliding your fingertips along the yardstick for as far as possible.

5. Do the test three times.
   Record your best score to the nearest inch: _____ inches
   The greater your reach, the higher your score will be, and the more flexible you are.

Determine Your Exercise Risk

You often hear that you should talk to your doctor before starting any exercise program, and we want to encourage you to do that. But if you're curious now, take this test as well. This quiz was adapted from the Physical Activity Readiness Questionnaire (PAR-Q) developed by the Canadian Society for Exercise Physiology to determine your exercise risk. This quiz is only applicable to people ages 15 to 69; anyone older than 69 *will* need to talk to his or her doctor no matter what.

Has your doctor ever said that you have a heart condition and that you should only do physical activity recommended by a doctor?

Yes _____   No _____

Do you feel pain in your chest when you do physical activity?

Yes _____   No _____

In the past month, have you had chest pain when you were not doing physical activity?

Yes _____   No _____

Do you lose your balance because of dizziness or do you ever lose consciousness?

Yes _____   No _____

Do you have a bone or joint problem (for example, back, knee or hip) that could be made worse by a change in your physical activity?

Yes _____   No _____

Is your doctor currently prescribing drugs (for example, water pills) for your blood pressure or heart condition?

Yes _____   No _____

Do you know of any other reason why you should not do physical activity?

Yes _____   No _____

If you answered YES to one or more questions

Consult with your doctor BEFORE you start becoming much more physically active or BEFORE you have a fitness appraisal. Tell your doctor about the PAR-Q and which questions you answered YES. You may be able to do any activity you want—as long as you start slowly and build up gradually. Or, you may need to restrict your activities to those that are safe for you. Talk with your doctor about the kinds of activities you wish to participate in and follow his or her advice.

If you answered NO to all questions

If you answered NO to all PAR-Q questions, you can be reasonably sure that you can:

Start becoming much more physically active—begin slowly and build up gradually. This is the safest and easiest way to go.

Take part in a fitness appraisal—this is an excellent way to determine your basic fitness so that you can plan the best way for you to live actively.

Can I test myself?

There are various tests you can do at home in private. Just make sure the test is FDA approved by checking the FDA's Web site at www.accessdata.fda.gov/scripts/cdrh/cfdocs/cfIVD/Search.cfm.

Here are the various tests that are available for home use.

Cholesterol

Diabetes

Fecal occult (blood in stool)

Menopause

Ovulation

Pregnancy

Urinary tract infection

Vaginal pH

But please know that no test is a substitute for your relationship with your doctor. You may have lots of information, but without the guidance of a trained medical professional, you may have no context for understanding or perspective on how to use that information.

Take the time to find a doctor you really connect with—in the best-case scenario, the doctor-patient relationship itself can be a part of your healing process.

Acknowledgments

From Jay McGraw, executive producer of The Doctors:

From day one, *The Doctors* has been committed to producing shows that are relevant, informative, and of the highest and best use of daily television. There are no greater stakes than managing your health, and *The Doctors* takes our responsibility to our viewers seriously: to investigate the latest medical information and present it in a way that is informative, relevant, and entertaining. Five days a week, real people with real health situations tune in to get real health and medical solutions in real time. *The Doctors* is dedicated to getting it right.

The Doctors 5-Minute Health Fixes has been a team effort with some of the industries' best and brightest contributing. First and foremost, *The Doctors'* deep appreciation goes to Dr. Phil McGraw for his relentless dedication to creating television that improves and impacts people's lives daily. You paved the way for us to do what we do.

Thanks to the heartbeat of *The Doctors:* Dr. Travis Stork, Dr. Lisa Masterson, Dr. Andrew Ordon, and Dr. Jim Sears. You bring the MD to TV. Your passion and commitment to the health concerns of millions is inspirational. And thanks to Carla Pennington and Andrew Scher, the brains and behind-the-scenes dream team, for your uncompromising commitment to bringing groundbreaking information to our viewers. Appreciation also goes to our entire team for helping to make *The Doctors* the Emmy Award–winning show that it is. And thank you to the best crew in television. We are just getting started.

We dedicate this book to our viewers because they are the inspiration behind everything that we do. Thank you for making *The Doctors* your trusted source for medical and health information.

In addition to relying on our own doctors' professional training and experiences for this book, we also consulted some of the most respected medical experts in their fields. A special thanks to Dwight Lundell, MD, board-certified cardiovascular surgeon with more than 30 years of experience and author of *The Cure for Heart Disease;* and G. Frank Lawlis, PhD, ABPP, a fellow of the American Psychological Association, chairman of the advisory board for the *Dr. Phil* show, and *New York Times* best-selling author of *ADD Answer* and *IQ Answer.*

Much appreciation also goes to Gary C. Morchower, MD, clinical professor of pediatrics at the University of Texas Southwestern Medical School and author of *1001 Healthy Baby Answers;* Bruce A. Phillips, MD, board-certified clinician in family medicine and founder of Park Cities Medical Associates with over 21 years of experience; Laura Blocker, MD, board-certified clinician in obstetrics and gynecology; and Marina Johnson, MD, FACE, board-certified endocrinologist with 28 years of clinical experience treating over 100,000 female patients, medical director of the Institute of Endocrinology and Preventive Medicine in the Dallas–Fort Worth Metroplex, and author of *Outliving Your Ovaries,* a guidebook for women to help evaluate the risks and benefits of hormone replacement therapy.

We want to thank our publishing partner Rodale for their commitment to making this book the "medical guide to reach for" in every home in America. We especially acknowledge Colin Dickerman and Mariska van Aalst for their contribution to this book, and Zach Martin for his help in designing the cover. Thanks to Dupree/Miller, who always bring an unwavering commitment to our projects. They are second to none. Thanks to Jan Miller, Shannon Marven, and Lacy Lynch.

This is the year my daughter arrived. Her mother and I are grateful beyond words for the happiness, joy, and love she brings to our lives. Also, thank you to my mom and dad for leading by example. And last but certainly the closest to my heart, thank you Erica for your endless love and support.

From Mariska van Aalst:

My tremendous thanks goes to Sara Vigneri, ace researcher and all-around fantastic person. Together, we owe huge thanks to Rodale—both the company and the family—which gave us both our start in health journalism. I'd also love to thank Colin Dickerman, for many insightful (and hilarious) conversations; Heather Jackson, for her dear friendship, creativity, and keen editorial eye; and Zachary Greenwald, the talented and tireless (and always cheerful) captain who kept this book on the tracks.

And, of course, thanks to the ever-patient Matthew, Téa, and Sabena—with immeasurable love and gratitude.

Selected References

Chapter One

American Academy of Periodontology. Tooth or Consequences: 10 Steps to Add Years to Your Life. March 9, 1999. http://www.perio.org/consumer/addyears.htm.

Centers for Disease Control and Prevention. Clinical Preventive Services. February 10, 2010. http://www.cdc.gov/Aging/services/index.htm.

Department of Health, United Kingdom. Small Change, Big Difference. February 8, 2007. http://www.dh.gov.uk/en/Publichealth/Healthimprovement/Smallchangebigdifference/DH_4134042.

Foster DP, Chua CT, Ungar LH. How Long Will I Live? n.d. http://gosset.wharton.upenn.edu/mortality/perl/CalcForm.html.

Fraser GE,Shavlik DJ. 2001. Ten Years of Life: Is It a Matter of Choice? *Arch Intern Med* 2001;161:1645–52.

Grassi D, Lippi C, Necozione S, Desideri G, Ferri C. Short-Term Administration of Dark Chocolate Is Followed by a Significant Increase in Insulin Sensitivity and a Decrease in Blood Pressure in Healthy Persons. *Am J Clin Nutr* 2005;81(3):611–4.

Harvard Medical School. Links to Resources for Creating a Personal Health Record. *Harv Heart Lett,* January 2009. http://www.health.harvard.edu/newsletters/Harvard_Heart_Letter/2009/January/Links-to-resources-for-creating-a-personal-health-record.

Koskimäki J, Shiri R, Tammela T, Häkkinen J, Hakama M, Auvinen A. Regular Intercourse Protects Against Erectile Dysfunction: Tampere Aging Male Urologic Study. *Am J Med* 2008;121(7):592–6.

Lloyd-Williams F, Mwatsama M, Ireland R, Capewell S. Small Changes in Snacking Behaviour: The Potential Impact on CVD Mortality. *Public Health Nutr* 2009;12(6):871–6.

Lopez-Garcia E, van Dam RM, Li TY, Rodriguez-Artalejo F, Hu FB. The Relationship of Coffee Consumption with Mortality. *Ann Intern Med* 2008;148:904–14.

Olshansky SJ, Passaro DJ, Hershow RC, Layden J, Carnes BA, Brody J, Hayflick L, Butler RN, Allison DB, Ludwig DS. A Potential Decline in Life Expectancy in the United States in the 21st Century. *N Engl J Med* 2005;352(11):1138–45.

Redelmeier DA, Bayoumi AM. Time Lost by Driving Fast in the United States. *Med Decis Making* 2010;30(3):E12–9 [Epub ahead of print].

Rodearmel SJ, Wyatt HR, Stroebele N, Smith SM, Ogden LG, Hill JO. Small Changes in Dietary Sugar and Physical Activity as an Approach to Preventing Excessive Weight Gain: The America on the Move Family Study. *Pediatrics* 2007;120(4):e869–79.

Smith A. Effects of Chewing Gum on Cognitive Function, Mood and Physiology in Stressed and Non-Stressed Volunteers. *Nutr Neurosci* 2010;13(1):7–16.

Davey Smith G, Frankel S, Yarnell J. Sex and Death: Are They Related? Findings from the Caerphilly Cohort Study. *BMJ* 1997;315(7123):1641–4.

Willcox BJ, He Q, Chen R, Yano K, Masaki KH, Grove JS, Donion TA, Willcox DC, Curb JD. Midlife Risk Factors and Healthy Survival in Men. *JAMA* 2006;296:2343–50.

Yates LB, Djoussé L, Kurth T, Buring JE, Gaziano JM. Exceptional Longevity in Men: Modifiable Factors Associated with Survival and Function to Age 90 Years. *Arch Intern Med* 2008;168(3):284–90.

Chapter Two

American Heart Association. Healthy Lifestyle. n.d. http://www.americanheart.org/presenter.jhtml?identifier=1200009.

American Heart Association. *The New American Heart Association Cookbook*. New York: Clarkson Potter, 1998.

Anonymous. Heart and Blood Vessel Disorders: High Blood Pressure. Merck Manuals Online Medical Library, April 2007. http://www.merck.com/mmhe/sec03/ch022/ch022a.html.

Baumhäkel M, Schlimmer N, Kratz MT, Böhm M. Erectile Dysfunction: Indicator of End-Organ Damage in Cardiovascular Patients. *Med Klin (Munich)* 2009;104(4):309–13.

Böhm M, Baumhäkel M, Teo K, Sleight P, Probstfield J, Gao P, Mann JF, Diaz R, Dagenais GR, Jennings GL, Liu L, Jansky P, Yusuf S, ONTARGET/TRANSCEND Erectile Dysfunction Substudy Investigators. Erectile Dysfunction Predicts Cardiovascular Events in High-Risk Patients Receiving Telmisartan, Ramipril, or Both: The ONgoing Telmisartan Alone and in combination with Ramipril Global Endpoint Trial/Telmisartan Randomized AssessmeNt Study in ACE iNtolerant subjects with cardiovascular Disease (ONTARGET/TRANSCEND) Trials. *Circulation* 2010;121(12):1439–46.

Brown L, Rosner B, Willett WW, Sacks FM. Cholesterol-Lowering Effects of Dietary Fiber: A Meta-Analysis. *Am J Clin Nutr* 1999;69(1):30–42.

Carnethon MR, Yan L, Greenland P, Garside DB, Dyer AR, Metzger B, Daviglus ML. Resting Heart Rate in Middle Age and Diabetes Development in Older Age. *Diabetes Care* 2008;31(2):335–9.

Carter TJ, Gilovich T. The Relative Relativity of Material and Experiential Purchases. *Soc Psychol* 2010;98(1):146–59.

Cheng M. Happiness Helps When It Comes to the Heart. Associated Press, February 18, 2010.

Davidson KW, Mostofsky E, Whang W. Don't Worry, Be Happy: Positive Affect and Reduced 10-Year Incident Coronary Heart Disease: The Canadian Nova Scotia Health Survey. *Eur Heart J* Feb 17, 2010 [Epub ahead of print].

Dunstan DW, Barr EL, Healy GN, Salmon J, Shaw JE, Balkau B, Magliano DJ, Cameron AJ, Zimmet PZ, Owen N. Television Viewing Time and Mortality: The Australian Diabetes, Obesity and Lifestyle Study (AusDiab). *Circulation* 2010;121(3):384–91.

Elliot WJ. Cyclic and Circadian Variations in Cardiovascular Events. *Am J Hypertens* 2001;14(9 Pt 2):291S–295S.

Elmas E, Kälsch T, Suvajac N, Leweling H. Activation of Coagulation During Alimentary Lipemia under Real-Life Conditions. *J Pers Int J Cardiol* 2007;114(2):172–5.

FamilyDoctor.org Editorial Staff. Blood Pressure Monitoring at Home. FamilyDoctor.org, November 2009. http://familydoctor.org/online/famdocen/home/common/heartdisease/treatment/128.html.

Farzaneh-Far R, Lin J, Epel ES, Harris WS, Blackburn EH, Whooley MA. Association of Marine Omega-3 Fatty Acid Levels with Telomeric Aging in Patients with Coronary Heart Disease. *JAMA* 2010;303(3):250–7.

Fox K, Ford I, Steg PG, Tendera M, Robertson M, Ferrari R. Heart Rate as a Prognostic Risk Factor in Patients with Coronary Artery Disease and Left-Ventricular Systolic Dysfunction (BEAUTIFUL): A Subgroup Analysis of a Randomised Controlled Trial. *Lancet* 2008;372(9641):817–21.

Grewen KM, Girdler SS, Amico J, Light KC. Effects of Partner Support on Resting Oxytocin, Cortisol, Norepinephrine, and Blood Pressure Before and After Warm Partner Contact. *Psychosom Med* 2005;67:531–8.

Haldar SM, Lu Y, Jeyaraj D, Kawanami D, Cui Y, Eapen SJ, Hao C, Li Y, Doughman YQ, Watanabe M, Shimizu K, Kuivaniemi H, Sadoshima J, Margulies KB, Cappola TP, Jain MK. Klf15 Deficiency Is a Molecular Link Between Heart Failure and Aortic Aneurysm Formation. *Sci Transl Med* 2010;2(26):26ra26.

Johns Hopkins Medicine. Heart Attack: Symptoms and Remedies. Johns Hopkins Health Alerts, n.d. http://www.johnshopkinshealthalerts.com/symptoms_remedies/heart_attack/83-1.html.

Kemper KJ, Gardiner P, Woods C. Changes in Use of Herbs and Dietary Supplements (HDS) among Clinicians Enrolled in an Online Curriculum. *BMC Complement Altern Med* 2007;7:21.

Khaw KT, Wareham N, Bingham S, Luben R, Welch A, Day N. Association of Hemoglobin A1c with Cardiovascular Disease and Mortality in Adults: The European Prospective Investigation into Cancer in Norfolk. *Ann Intern Med* 2004;141(6):413–20.

Klabunde RE. *Cardiovascular Physiology Concepts*. Philadelphia: Lippincott Williams and Wilkins, 2004.

Lab Tests Online. Lipid Profile. January 4, 2009. http://www.labtestsonline.org/understanding/analytes/lipid/glance-5.html.

Ladenson PW, Kristensen JD, Ridgway EC, Olsson AG, Carlsson B, Klein I, Baxter JD, Angelin B. Use of the Thyroid Hormone Analogue Eprotirome in Statin-Treated Dyslipidemia. *N Engl J Med* 2010;362(10):906–16.

Light KC, Grewen KM, Amico JA. More Frequent Partner Hugs and Higher Oxytocin Levels Are Linked to Lower Blood Pressure and Heart Rate in Premenopausal Women. *Biol Psychol* 2005;69(1):5–21.

Lopez-Garcia E, van Dam RM, Li TY, Rodriguez-Artalejo F, Hu FB. The Relationship of Coffee Consumption with Mortality. *Ann Intern Med* 2008;148(12):904–14.

Medline Plus. Health Topics: Heart Diseases. February 7, 2010. http://www.nlm.nih.gov/medlineplus/heartdiseases.html.

Montana State University–Bozeman. Physiology and Psychology: Cardiovascular Factors. April 1998. http://btc.montana.edu/olympics/physiology/cf01.html.

Moyer AE, Rodin J, Grilo CM, Cummings N, Larson LM, Rebuffé-Scrive M. Stress-Induced Cortisol Response and Fat Distribution in Women. *Obes Res* 1994;2(3):255–62.

National Heart Lung and Blood Institute. How the Heart Works. National Heart Lung and Blood Institute, Diseases and Conditions Index, July 2009. http://www.nhlbi.nih.gov/health/dci/Diseases/hhw/hhw_whatis.html.

Natural Standard Research Collaboration. Omega-3 Fatty Acids, Fish Oil, Alpha-Linolenic Acid. Mayoclinic.com, February 1, 2010. http://www.mayoclinic.com/health/fish-oil/NS_patient-fishoil.

Nawijn J, Marchand MA, Veenhoven R, Vingerhoets AJ. Vacationers Happier, but Most Not Happier after a Holiday. *Appl Res Qual Life* 2010;5(1):35–47.

Palar K, Sturm R. Potential Societal Savings from Reduced Sodium Consumption in the U.S. Adult Population. *Am J Health Promot* 2009;24(1):49–57.

Ricketts ML, Boekschoten MV, Kreeft AJ, Hooiveld GJ, Moen CJ, Müller M, Frants RR, Kasanmoentalib S, Post SM, Princen HM, Porter JG, Katan MB, Hofker MH, Moore DD. The Cholesterol-Raising Factor from Coffee Beans, Cafestol, as an Agonist Ligand for the Farnesoid and Pregnane X Receptors. *Mol Endocrinol* 2007;21(7):1603–16.

Roerecke M, Rehm J. Irregular Heavy Drinking Occasions and Risk of Ischemic Heart Disease: A Systematic Review and Meta-Analysis. *Am J Epidemiol* 2010;171(6):633–44.

Saunders E. High Blood Pressure: Tips to Stop the Silent Killer. University of Maryland Medical Center, August 7, 2008. http://www.umm.edu/features/blood_pressure.htm.

Selvin E, Steffes MW, Zhu H, Matsushita K, Wagenknecht L, Pankow J, Coresh J, Brancati FL. Glycated Hemoglobin, Diabetes, and Cardiovascular Risk in Nondiabetic Adults. *N Engl J Med* 2010;362(9):800–11.

Sherwood L. *Human Physiology: From Cells to Systems*. Belmont, CA: Brooks Cole, 2007. p. 336.

Sieri S, Krogh V, Berrino F, Evangelista A, Agnoli C, Brighenti F, Pellegrini N, Palli D, Masala G, Sacerdote C, Veglia F, Tumino R, Frasca G, Grioni S, Pala V, Mattiello A, Chiodini P, Panico S. Dietary Glycemic Load and Index and Risk of Coronary Heart Disease in a Large Italian Cohort: The EPICOR Study. *Arch Intern Med* 2010;170(7):640–7.

Stampfer MJ, Hu FB, Manson JE, Rimm EB, Willett WC. Primary Prevention of Coronary Heart Disease in Women through Diet and Lifestyle. *N Engl J Med* 2000;343(1):16–22.

Urgert R, Schulz AG, Katan MB. Effects of Cafestol and Kahweol from Coffee Grounds on Serum Lipids and Serum Liver Enzymes in Humans. *Am J Clin Nutr* 1995;61(1):149–54.

Chapter Three

Birns J, Morris R, Jarosz J, Markus HS, Kalra L. Hypertension-Related Cognitive Decline: Is the Time Right for Intervention Studies? *Minerva Cardioangiol* 2009;57(6):813–30.

Born J, Wagner U. Memory Consolidation During Sleep: Role of Cortisol Feedback. *Ann N Y Acad Sci* 2004;1032:198–201.

Boyle PA, Buchman AS, Barnes LL, Bennett DA. Effect of a Purpose in Life on Risk of Incident Alzheimer Disease and Mild Cognitive Impairment in Community-Dwelling Older Persons. *Arch Gen Psychiatry* 2010;67(3):304–10.

Brody J. Even More Reasons to Get a Move On. *New York Times,* March 1, 2010.

Cortés B, Núñez I, Cofán M, Gilabert R, Pérez-Heras A, Casals E, Deulofeu R, Ros E. Acute Effects of High-Fat Meals Enriched with Walnuts or Olive Oil on Postprandial Endothelial Function. *J Am Coll Cardiol* 2006;48(8):1666–71.

Davidson RJ, Kabat-Zinn J, Schumacher J, Rosenkranz M, Muller D, Santorelli SF, Urbanowski F, Harrington A, Bonus K, Sheridan JF. Alterations in Brain and Immune Function Produced by Mindfulness Meditation. *Psychosom Med* 2003;65(4):564–70.

Dubinski A, Zdrojewicz Z. [The Role of Interleukin-6 in Development and Progression of Atherosclerosis]. *Pol Merkur Lekarski* 2007;22(130):291–4.

Dunstan DW, Barr EL, Healy GN, Salmon J, Shaw JE, Balkau B, Magliano DJ, Cameron AJ, Zimmet PZ, Owen N. Television Viewing Time and Mortality: The Australian Diabetes, Obesity and Lifestyle Study (AusDiab). *Circulation* 2010;121(3):384–91.

Familydoctor.org Editorial Staff. Head Injuries: What to Watch for Afterward. American Academy of Family Physicians, October 2009. http://familydoctor.org/online/famdocen/home/common/brain/head/084.html.

Fontana L, Eagon JC, Trujillo ME, Scherer PE, Klein S. Visceral Fat Adipokine Secretion Is Associated with Systemic Inflammation in Extremely Obese Humans. *Diabetes* 2007;56:1010–3.

Grossman P, Niemann L, Schmidt S, Walach H. Mindfulness-Based Stress Reduction and Health Benefits: A Meta-Analysis. *J Psychosom Res* 2004;57(1):35–43.

Gu Y, Nieves JW, Stern Y, Luchsinger JA, Scarmeas N. Food Combination and Alzheimer Disease Risk: A Protective Diet. *Arch Neurol* 2010;67(6) [Epub ahead of print].

Hairston KG, Bryer-Ash M, Norris JM, Haffner S, Bowden DW, Wagenknecht LE. Sleep Duration and Five-Year Abdominal Fat Accumulation in a Minority Cohort: The IRAS Family Study. *Sleep* 2010;33(3):289–95.

Honjo K, van Reekum R, Verhoeff NP. Alzheimer's Disease and Infection: Do Infectious Agents Contribute to Progression of Alzheimer's Disease? *Alzheimers Dement* 2009;5(4):348–60.

Kiecolt-Glaser JK, Christian L, Preston H, Houts CR, Malarkey WB, Emery CF, Glaser R. Stress, Inflammation, and Yoga Practice. *Psychosom Med* 2010;72(2):113–21.

Kristiansen OP, Mandrup-Poulsen T. Interleukin-6 and Diabetes: The Good, the Bad, or the Indifferent? *Diabetes* 2005;54 Suppl 2:S114–24.

Kuller LH, Margolis KL, Gaussoin SA, Bryan NR, Kerwin D, Limacher M, Wassertheil-Smoller S, Williamson J, Robinson JG. Relationship of Hypertension, Blood Pressure, and Blood Pressure Control with White Matter Abnormalities in the Women's Health Initiative Memory Study (WHIMS)-MRI Trial. *J Clin Hypertens (Greenwich)* 2010;12(3):203–12.

Lautenschlager NT, Cox KL, Flicker L, Foster JK, van Bockxmeer FM, Xiao J, Greenop KR, Almeida OP. Effect of Physical Activity on Cognitive Function in Older Adults at Risk for Alzheimer Disease: A Randomized Trial. *JAMA* 2008;300(9):1027–37.

Levitan EB, Yang AZ, Wolk A, Mittleman MA. Adiposity and Incidence of Heart Failure Hospitalization and Mortality: A Population-Based Prospective Study. *Circ Heart Fail* 2009;2(3):202–8.

Levy SB. Antibacterial Household Products: Cause for Concern. *Emerg Infect Dis* 2001;7(3 Suppl):512–5.

Liu-Ambrose T, Nagamatsu LS, Graf P, Beattie BL, Ashe MC, Handy TC. Resistance Training and Executive Functions: A 12-Month Randomized Controlled Trial. *Arch Intern Med* 2010;170(2):170–8.

Mander BA, Colecchia E, Spiegel KS, Van Cauter E. Short Sleep: A Risk Factor for Insulin Resistance and Obesity. *Sleep* 2001;24(Suppl):A74–5.

Manjunath NK, Telles S. Spatial and Verbal Memory Test Scores following Yoga and Fine Arts Camps for School Children. *Indian J Physiol Pharmacol* 2004;48(3):353–6.

Marangoni F, Colombo C, Martiello A, Poli A, Paoletti R, Galli C. Levels of the n-3 Fatty Acid Eicosapentaenoic Acid in Addition to Those of Alpha Linolenic Acid Are Significantly Raised in Blood Lipids by the Intake of Four Walnuts a Day in Humans. *Nutr Metab Cardiovasc Dis* 2007;17(6):457–61.

Mednick S, Nakayama K, Stickgold R. Sleep-Dependent Learning: A Nap Is as Good as a Night. *Nat Neurosci* 2003;6(7):697–8.

Mori H, Yamamoto H, Kuwashima M, Saito S, Ukai H, Hirao K, Yamauchi M, Umemura S. How Does Deep Breathing Affect Office Blood Pressure and Pulse Rate? *Hypertens Res* 2005;28(6):499–504.

Neylan TC, Schuff N, Lenoci M, Yehuda R, Weiner MW, Marmar CR. Cortisol Levels Are Positively Correlated with Hippocampal *N*-Acetylaspartate. *Biol Psychiatry* 2003;54(10):1118–21.

Pajonk FG, Wobrock T, Gruber O, Scherk H, Berner D, Kaizl I, Kierer A, Müller S, Oest M, Meyer T, Backens M, Schneider-Axmann T, Thornton AE, Honer WG, Falkai P. Hippocampal Plasticity in Response to Exercise in Schizophrenia. *Arch Gen Psychiatry* 2010;67(2):133–43.

Peterson JM. Left-Handedness: Differences between Student Artists and Scientists. *Percept Mot Skills* 1979;48(3 Pt 1):961–2.

Robert McComb JJ, Tacon A, Randolph P, Caldera Y. A Pilot Study to Examine the Effects of a Mindfulness-Based Stress-Reduction and Relaxation Program on Levels of Stress Hormones, Physical Functioning, and Submaximal Exercise Responses. *J Altern Complement Med* 2004;10(5):819–27.

Rothwell PM, Howard SC, Dolan E, O'Brien E, Dobson JE, Dahlöf B, Sever PS, Poulter NR. Prognostic Significance of Visit-to-Visit Variability, Maximum Systolic Blood Pressure, and Episodic Hypertension. *Lancet* 2010;375(9718):895–905.

Sattelmair JR, Kurth T, Buring JE, Lee IM. Physical Activity and Risk of Stroke in Women. *Stroke* Apr 6, 2010 [Epub ahead of print].

Shenhar-Tsarfaty S, Ben Assayag E, Bova I, Shopin L, Fried M, Berliner S, Shapira I, Bornstein NM. Interleukin-6 as an Early Predictor for One-Year Survival Following an Ischaemic Stroke/Transient Ischaemic Attack. *Int J Stroke* 2010;5(1):16–20.

Small GW, Moody TD, Siddarth P, Bookheimer SY. Your Brain on Google: Patterns of Cerebral Activation during Internet Searching. *Am J Geriatr Psychiatry* 2009;17(2):116–26.

Smith A. Effects of Chewing Gum on Cognitive Function, Mood and Physiology in Stressed and Non-Stressed Volunteers. *Nutr Neurosci* 2010;13(1):7–16.

Tang YY, Ma Y, Wang J, Fan Y, Feng S, Lu Q, Yu Q, Sui D, Rothbart MK, Fan M, Posner MI. Short-Term Meditation Training Improves Attention and Self-Regulation. *Proc Natl Acad Sci U S A* 2007;104(43):17152–6.

Wagner D, Manahilov V, Loffler G, Gordon GE, Dutton GN. Visual Noise Selectively Degrades Vision in Migraine. *Invest Ophthalmol Vis Sci* 2010;51(4):2294–9.

Wersching H, Duning T, Lohmann H, Mohammadi S, Stehling C, Fobker M, Conty M, Minnerup J, Ringelstein EB, Berger K, Deppe M, Knecht S. Serum C-Reactive Protein Is Linked to Cerebral Microstructural Integrity and Cognitive Function. *Neurology* 2010;74(13):1022–9.

Winter Y, Rohrmann S, Linseisen J, Lanczik O, Ringleb PA, Hebebrand J, Back T. Contribution of Obesity and Abdominal Fat Mass to Risk of Stroke and Transient Ischemic Attacks. *Stroke* 2008;39(12):3145–51.

Wu SD, Lo PC. Inward-Attention Meditation Increases Parasympathetic Activity: A Study Based on Heart Rate Variability. *Biomed Res* 2008;29(5):245–50.

Chapter Four

Centers for Disease Control and Prevention. Prevention of Pneumococcal Disease: Recommendations of the Advisory Committee on Immunization Practices (ACIP). *MMWR Recomm Rep* 1997;46(RR-8):1–24.

Doll R, Peto R, Boreham J, Sutherland I. Mortality in Relation to Smoking: 50 Years' Observations on Male British Doctors. *BMJ* 2004;328(7455):1519.

Foster GD, Borradaile KE, Sanders MH, Millman R, Zammit G, Newman AB, Wadden TA, Kelley D, Wing RR, Pi-Sunyer FX, Reboussin D, Kuna ST, Sleep AHEAD Research Group of Look AHEAD Research Group. A Randomized Study on the Effect of Weight Loss on Obstructive Sleep Apnea among Obese Patients with Type 2 Diabetes: The Sleep AHEAD Study. *Arch Intern Med* 2009;169(17):1619–26.

Kassel JC, King D, Spurling GK. Saline Nasal Irrigation for Acute Upper Respiratory Tract Infections. *Cochrane Database Syst Rev* 2010;17(3):CD006821.

Kirshner M. Preliminary Exploration of Online Social Support among Adults with Asthma. *AMIA Annu Symp Proc* 2003;2003:895.

Midoro-Horiuti T, Tiwari R, Watson CS, Goldblum RM. Maternal Bisphenol A Exposure Promotes the Development of Experimental Asthma in Mouse Pups. *Environ Health Perspect* 2010;118(2):273–7.

National Institute on Deafness and Other Communication Disorders. Smell Disorders. July 2009. http://www.nidcd.nih.gov/health/smelltaste/smell.asp.

Oraka E, King ME, Callahan DB. Asthma and Serious Psychological Distress: Prevalence and Risk Factors among US Adults, 2001-2007. *Chest* 2010;137(3):609–16.

Paul IM, Beiler J, McMonagle A, Shaffer ML, Duda L, Berlin CM Jr. Effect of Honey, Dextromethorphan, and No Treatment on Nocturnal Cough and Sleep Quality for Coughing Children and Their Parents. *Arch Pediatr Adolesc Med* 2007;161(12):1140–6.

Schnoll RA, Patterson F, Wileyto EP, Heitjan DF, Shields AE, Asch DA, Lerman C. Effectiveness of Extended-Duration Transdermal Nicotine Therapy: A Randomized Trial. *Ann Intern Med* 2010; 152(3):144–51.

Shimazu T, Inoue M, Sasazuki S, Iwasaki M, Sawada N, Yamaji T, Tsugane S. Isoflavone Intake and Risk of Lung Cancer: A Prospective Cohort Study in Japan. *Am J Clin Nutr* 2010;91(3):722–8.

Varraso R, Willett WC, Camargo CA Jr. Prospective Study of Dietary Fiber and Risk of Chronic Obstructive Pulmonary Disease among US Women and Men. *Am J Epidemiol* 2010;171(7):776–84.

Chapter Five

American Heart Association. Drinking Sugar-Sweetened Beverages Daily Linked to Diabetes, Cardiovascular Disease, Increased Healthcare Costs: Abstract P365. March 5, 2010. http://www.newsroom.heart.org/index.php?s=43&item=976 [news release].

Belkaid A, Currie JC, Desgagnés J, Annabi B. The Chemopreventive Properties of Chlorogenic Acid Reveal a Potential New Role for the Microsomal Glucose-6-Phosphate Translocase in Brain Tumor Progression. *Cancer Cell Int* 2006;6:7.

Bouchard MF, Bellinger DC, Wright RO, Weisskopf MG. Attention-Deficit/Hyperactivity Disorder and Urinary Metabolites of Organophosphate Pesticides. *Pediatrics* May 17, 2010 [Epub ahead of print].

Chandalia M, Garg A, Lutjohann D, von Bergmann K, Grundy SM, Brinkley LJ. Beneficial Effects of High Dietary Fiber Intake in Patients with Type 2 Diabetes Mellitus. *N Engl J Med* 2000;342(19):1392–8.

Clean Air Council. Waste Reduction and Recycling: Waste Facts and Figures. n.d. http://www.cleanair.org/Waste/wasteFacts.html.

Conceição de Oliveira M, Sichieri R, Sanchez Moura A. Weight Loss Associated with a Daily Intake of Three Apples or Three Pears among Overweight Women. *Nutrition* 2003;19(3):253–6.

de Vrese M. Health Benefits of Probiotics and Prebiotics in Women. *Menopause Int* 2009;15(1):35–40.

de Vrese M, Schrezenmeir J. Probiotics, Prebiotics, and Synbiotics. *Adv Biochem Eng Biotechnol* 2008;111:1–66.

Di Stefano M, Micelli E, Gotti S, Missanelli A, Mazzocchi S, Corazza GR. The Effect of Oral Alpha-Galactosidase on Intestinal Gas Production and Gas-Related Symptoms. *Dig Dis Sci* 2007;52(1):78–83.

Dominguez-Bello MG, Blaser MJ. Do You Have a Probiotic in Your Future? *Microbes Infect* 2008;10(9):1072–6.

Fasano A, Berti I, Gerarduzzi T, Not T, Colletti RB, Drago S, Elitsur Y, Green PHR, Guandalini S, Hill ID, Pietzak M, Ventura A, Thorpe M, Kryszak D, Fornaroli F, Wasserman SS, Murray JA, Horvath K. Prevalence of Celiac Disease in At-Risk and Not-at-Risk Groups in the United States: A Large Multicenter Study. *Arch Intern Med* 2003;163(3):268–92.

Fass R, Quan SF, O'Connor GT, Ervin A, Iber C. Predictors of Heartburn During Sleep in a Large Prospective Cohort Study. *Chest* 2005;127(5):1658–66.

Fernando GR, Martha RM, Evangelina R. Consumption of Soft Drinks with Phosphoric Acid as a Risk Factor for the Development of Hypocalcemia in Postmenopausal Women. *J Clin Epidemiol* 1999;52(10):1007–10.

Furne JK, Levitt MD. Factors Influencing Frequency of Flatus Emission by Healthy Subjects. *Dig Dis Sci* 1996;41(8):1631–5.

Ganiats TG, Norcross WA, Halverson AL, Burford PA, Palinkas LA. Does Beano Prevent Gas? A Double-Blind Crossover Study of Oral Alpha-Galactosidase to Treat Dietary Oligosaccharide Intolerance. *J Fam Pract* 1994;39(5):441–5.

Gordon MH, Wishart K. Effects of Chlorogenic Acid and Bovine Serum Albumin on the Oxidative Stability of Low Density Lipoproteins in Vitro. *J Agric Food Chem* 2010;58(9):5828–33.

Hastert TA, Babey SH. School Lunch Source and Adolescent Dietary Behavior. *Prev Chronic Dis* 2009;6(4):A117.

Isolauri E; Salminen S; Nutrition, Allergy, Mucosal Immunology, and Intestinal Microbiota (NAMI) Research Group. Probiotics: Use in Allergic Disorders: A Nutrition, Allergy, Mucosal Immunology, and Intestinal Microbiota (NAMI) Research Group Report. *J Clin Gastroenterol* 2008;42 Suppl 2:S91–6.

Isolauri E, Sütas Y, Kankaanpää P, Arvilommi H, Salminen S. Probiotics: Effects on Immunity. *Am J Clin Nutr* 2001;73(2 Suppl):444S–450S.

Jackson LP. Administrator Lisa P. Jackson, Remarks to the Commonwealth Club of San Francisco, as Prepared. September 29, 2009. http://yosemite.epa.gov/opa/admpress.nsf/a883dc3da7094f97852572a00065d7d8/fc4e2a 8c05343b3285257640007081c5.

Jain P, Nihill P, Sobkowski J, Agustin MZ. Commercial Soft Drinks: pH and in Vitro Dissolution of Enamel. *Gen Dent* 2007;55(2):150–4.

Kaltenbach T, Crockett S, Gerson LB. Are Lifestyle Measures Effective in Patients with Gastroesophageal Reflux Disease? An Evidence-Based Approach. *Arch Intern Med* 2006;166(9):965–71.

Katz LC, Just R, Castell DO. Body Position Affects Recumbent Postprandial Reflux. *J Clin Gastroenterol* 1994;18(4):280–3.

Kumar M, Kumar A, Nagpal R, Mohania D, Behare P, Verma V, Kumar P, Poddar D, Aggarwal PK, Henry CJ, Jain S, Yadav H. Cancer-Preventing Attributes of Probiotics: An Update. *Int J Food Sci Nutr* February 26, 2010 [Epub ahead of print].

Lawrence Hall of Science, University of California, Berkeley. Sugar Sleuths: Explorations for Parents and Their Children Ages 8–12. March 31, 2009. http://lawrencehallofscience.org/familyhealth/activities/sugarsleuths/ sugarsleuths.html.

Lin J, Curhan GC. Associations of Sweetened Beverages with Kidney Function Decline. Paper presented at the American Society of Nephrology 42nd Annual Meeting, San Diego, October 31, 2009.

Meng X, Zhang H, Law J, Tsang R, Tsang T. Detection of *Helicobacter pylori* from Food Sources by a Novel Multiplex PCR Assay. *J Food Saf* 2008;28(4):609–19.

Nojkov B, Rubenstein JH, Chey WD, Hoogerwerf WA. The Impact of Rotating Shift Work on the Prevalence of Irritable Bowel Syndrome in Nurses. *Am J Gastroenterol* 2010;105(4):842–7.

Okada H, Kuhn C, Feillet H, Bach J-F. The "Hygiene Hypothesis" for Autoimmune and Allergic Diseases: An Update. *Clin Exp Immunol* 2010;160(1):1–9.

Reyna-Villasmil N, Bermúdez-Pirela V, Mengual-Moreno E, Arias N, Cano-Ponce C, Leal-Gonzalez E, Souki A, Inglett GE, Israili ZH, Hernández-Hernández R, Valasco M, Arraiz N. Oat-Derived ß-Glucan Significantly Improves HDLC and Diminishes LDLC and Non-HDL Cholesterol in Overweight Individuals with Mild Hypercholesterolemia. *Am J Ther* 2007;14(2):203–12.

Rohsenow DJ, Howland J, Arnedt JT, Almeida AB, Greece J, Minsky S, Kempler CS, Sales S. 2010. Intoxication with Bourbon versus Vodka: Effects on Hangover, Sleep, and Next-Day Neurocognitive Performance in Young Adults. *Alcohol Clin Exp Res* 2010;34(3):509–18.

Salminen S, Nybom S, Meriluoto J, Collado MC, Vesterlund S, El-Nezami H. Interaction of Probiotics and Pathogens—Benefits to Human Health? *Curr Opin Biotechnol* 2010;21(2):157–67.

Sanders ME. Clinical Use of Probiotics: What Physicians Need to Know. *Am Fam Physician* 2008;78(9):1026.

Satyanarayana MN. Capsaicin and Gastric Ulcers. *Crit Rev Food Sci Nutr* 2006;46(4):275–328.

Savino F, Pelle E, Palumeri E, Oggero R, Miniero R. *Lactobacillus reuteri* (American Type Culture Collection Strain 55730) versus Simethicone in the Treatment of Infantile Colic: A Prospective Randomized Study. *Pediatrics* 2007;119(1):e124–30.

Schlosser, Eric. *Fast Food Nation.* New York: Houghton Mifflin, 2001.

Shoham DA, Durazo-Arvizu R, Kramer H, Luke A, Vupputuri S, Kshirsagar A, Cooper RS. Sugary Soda Consumption and Albuminuria: Results from the National Health and Nutrition Examination Survey, 1999–2004. *PLoS One* 2008;3(10):e3431.

Solomons NW, Vettorazzi L, Grazioso C. Use of an Oral Alpha-Galactosidase to Control Gastrointestinal Symptoms from Legume Oligosaccharides in Bean-Intolerant Subjects: A Doubly Masked, Controlled Therapeutic Trial. *Clin Res* 1991;39(Suppl):428A.

Stamatova I, Meurman JH. Probiotics: Health Benefits in the Mouth. *Am J Dent* 2009;22(6):329–38.

Steck SE, Gaudet MM, Eng SM, Britton JA, Teitelbaum SL, Neugut AI, Santella RM, Gammon MD. Cooked Meat and Risk of Breast Cancer—Lifetime versus Recent Dietary Intake. *Epidemiology* 2007;18(3):373–82.

Tran T, Lowry AM, El-Serag HB. Meta-Analysis: The Efficacy of Over-the-Counter Gastro-Oesophageal Reflux Disease Therapies. *Aliment Pharmacol Ther* 2007;25(2):143–53.

Tubelius P, Stan V, Zachrisson A. Increasing Work-Place Healthiness with the Probiotic *Lactobacillus reuteri*: A Randomised, Double-Blind Placebo-Controlled Study. *Environ Health* 2005;4:25. http://www.ehjournal.net/content/4/1/25.

Vanderpool C, Yan F, Polk DB. Mechanisms of Probiotic Action: Implications for Therapeutic Applications in Inflammatory Bowel Diseases. *Inflamm Bowel Dis* 2008;14(11):1585–96.

van Loo IH, Diederen BM, Savelkoul PH, Woudenberg JH, Roosendaal R, van Belkum A, Lemmens-den Toom N, Verhulst C, van Keulen PH, Kluytmans JA. Methicillin-Resistant *Staphylococcus aureus* in Meat Products, the Netherlands. *Emerg Infect Dis* 2007;13(11):1753–5.

Whitaker BD, Stommel JR. Distribution of Hydroxycinnamic Acid Conjugates in Fruit of Commercial Eggplant (*Solanum melongena* L.) Cultivars. *J Agric Food Chem* 2003;51(11):3448–54.

Chapter Six

Chung KT, Wong TY, Wei CI, Huang YW, Lin Y. Tannins and Human Health: A Review. *Crit Rev Food Sci Nutr* 1998;38(6):421–64.

Courteix D, Lespessailles E, Jaffre C, Obert P, Benhamou CL. Bone Material Acquisition and Somatic Development in Highly Trained Girl Gymnasts. *Acta Paediatr* 1999;88(8):803–8.

Devine A, Criddle RA, Dick IM, Kerr DA, Prince RL. A Longitudinal Study of the Effect of Sodium and Calcium Intakes on Regional Bone Density in Postmenopausal Women. *Am J Clin Nutr* 1995;62(4):740–5.

Fiss EM, Rule KL, Vikesland PJ. Formation of Chloroform and Other Chlorinated Byproducts by Chlorination of Triclosan-Containing Antibacterial Products. *Environ Sci Technol* 2007;41(7):2387–94.

Foran CM, Bennett ER, Benson WH. Developmental Evaluation of a Potential Non-Steroidal Estrogen: Triclosan. *Mar Environ Res* 2000;50(1–5):153–6.

Hong WH, Lee YH, Chen HC, Pei YC, Wu CY. Influence of Heel Height and Shoe Insert on Comfort Perception and Biomechanical Performance of Young Female Adults During Walking. *Foot Ankle Int* 2005;26(12):1042–8.

Martin LG, Freedman VA, Schoeni RF, Andreski PM. Trends in Disability and Related Chronic Conditions among People Ages Fifty to Sixty-Four. *Health Aff (Millwood)* 2010;29(4):725–31.

National Center for Chronic Disease Prevention and Health Promotion, Centers for Disease Control and Prevention. Fact Sheet: Adolescents and Young Adults. *Physical Activity and Health: A Report of the Surgeon General*. Rockville, MD: US Department of Health and Human Services, Office of the Surgeon General, 1999. http://www.cdc.gov/nccdphp/sgr/adoles.htm.

O'Hehir TE, Suvan JE. Dry Brushing Lingual Surfaces First. *J Am Dent Assoc* 1998;129(5):614.

Shakoor N, Block JA. Walking Barefoot Decreases Loading on the Lower Extremity Joints in Knee Osteoarthritis. *Arthritis Rheum* 2006;54(9):2923–7.

Shakoor N, Sengupta M, Foucher KC, Wimmer MA, Fogg LF, Block JA. The Effects of Common Footwear on Joint Loading in Osteoarthritis of the Knee. *Arthritis Care Res (Hoboken)* Feb 26, 2010 [Epub ahead of print].

Siegfried DR. Carpal Tunnel Relief: Wiggle While You Work. *Arthritis Today* n.d. http://www.arthritistoday.org/daily-living/relationships/on-the-job/carpal-tunnel-relief.php.

US Department of Health and Human Services. Determinants of Bone Health. In *Bone Health and Osteoporosis: A Report of the Surgeon General*. Rockville, MD: US Department of Health and Human Services, Office of the Surgeon General, 2004. http://www.surgeongeneral.gov/library/bonehealth/chapter_6.html.

Ward KA, Roberts SA, Adams JE, Mughal MZ. Bone Geometry and Density in the Skeleton of Pre-Pubertal Gymnasts and School Children. *Bone* 2005;36(6):1012–8.

Chapter Seven

American College of Obstetricians and Gynecologists, Committee on Gynecologic Practice. ACOG Committee Opinion #322: Compounded Bioidentical Hormones. *Obstet Gynecol* 2005;106(5 Pt 1):1139–40.

Apter D, Reinilä M, Vihko R. Some Endocrine Characteristics of Early Menarche, a Risk Factor for Breast Cancer, Are Preserved into Adulthood. *Int J Cancer* 1989;44(5):783–7.

Barbieri M, Gambardella A, Paolisso G, Varricchio M. Metabolic Aspects of the Extreme Longevity. *Exp Gerontol* 2008;43(2):74–8.

Berk LS, Felten DL, Tan SA, Bittman BB, Westengard J. Modulation of Neuroimmune Parameters during the Eustress of Humor-Associated Mirthful Laughter. *Altern Ther Health Med* 2001;7(2):62–76.

Berk LS, Tan SA, Berk D. Cortisol and Catecholamine Stress Hormone Decrease Is Associated with the Behavior of Perceptual Anticipation of Mirthful Laughter. *FASEB J* 2008;22:946.11.

Bray MS, Tsai JY, Villegas-Montoya C, Boland BB, Blasier Z, Egbejimi O, Kueht M, Young ME. Time-of-Day-Dependent Dietary Fat Consumption Influences Multiple Cardiometabolic Syndrome Parameters in Mice. *Int J Obes (Lond)* Mar 30, 2010 [Epub ahead of print].

Centers for Disease Control and Prevention. Chronic Disease Prevention and Health Promotion: Diabetes: Successes and Opportunities for Population-Based Prevention and Control: At a Glance 2010. April 8, 2010. http://www.cdc.gov/chronicdisease/resources/publications/aag/ddt.htm.

Duffey KJ, Gordon-Larsen P, Shikany JM, Guilkey D, Jacobs DR Jr, Popkin BM. Food Price and Diet and Health Outcomes: 20 Years of the CARDIA Study. *Arch Intern Med* 2010;170(5):420–6.

Franklin Institute. The Human Brain: Renew—Stress on the Brain. Resources for Science Learning, n.d. http://www.fi.edu/learn/brain/stress.html.

Fugh-Berman A, Bythrow J. Bioidentical Hormones for Menopausal Hormone Therapy: Variation on a Theme. *J Gen Intern Med* 2007;22(7):1030–4.

Gates MA, Tworoger SS, Eliassen AH, Missmer SA, Hankinson SE. Analgesic Use and Sex Steroid Hormone Concentrations in Postmenopausal Women. *Cancer Epidemiol Biomarkers Prev* 2010;19(4):1033–41.

Jenab M, Bueno-de-Mesquita HB, Ferrari P, van Duijnhoven FJ, Norat T, Pischon T, Jansen EH, Slimani N, Byrnes G, Rinaldi S, Tjønneland A, Olsen A, Overvad K, Boutron-Ruault MC, Clavel-Chapelon F, Morois S, Kaaks R, Linseisen J, Boeing H, Bergmann MM, Trichopoulou A, Misirli G, Trichopoulos D, Berrino F, Vineis P, Panico S, Palli D, Tumino R, Ros MM, van Gils CH, Peeters PH, Brustad M, Lund E, Tormo MJ, Ardanaz E, Rodríguez L, Sánchez MJ, Dorronsoro M, Gonzalez CA, Hallmans G, Palmqvist R, Roddam A, Key TJ, Khaw KT, Autier P, Hainaut P, Riboli E. Association Between Pre-Diagnostic Circulating Vitamin D Concentration and Risk of Colorectal Cancer in European Populations: A Nested Case-Control Study. *BMJ* 2010;340:b5500.

Kirkham S, Akilen R, Sharma S, Tsiami A. The Potential of Cinnamon to Reduce Blood Glucose Levels in Patients with Type 2 Diabetes and Insulin Resistance. *Diabetes Obes Metab* 2009;11(12):1100–13.

Kumar J, Muntner P, Kaskel FJ, Hailpern SM, Melamed ML. Prevalence and Associations of 25-Hydroxyvitamin D Deficiency in US Children: NHANES 2001-2004. *Pediatrics* 2009;124(3):e362–70.

Melzer D, Rice N, Depledge MH, Henley WE, Galloway TS. Association between Serum Perfluorooctanoic Acid (PFOA) and Thyroid Disease in the U.S. National Health and Nutrition Examination Survey. *Environ Health Perspect* 2010;118(5):686–92.

Mettler S, Schwarz I, Colombani PC. Additive Postprandial Blood Glucose-Attenuating and Satiety-Enhancing Effect of Cinnamon and Acetic Acid. *Nutr Res* 2009;29(10):723–7.

Mitchell D. Vitamin D Levels Inadequate in 70 Percent of U.S. Children: Improved Diet, Supplements, Sun Exposure among Remedial Options. *AAFP News Now*, August 18, 2009. http://www.aafp.org/online/en/home/publications/news/news-now/health-of-the-public/20090818vit-d.html.

Olshansky SJ, Passaro DJ, Hershow RC, Layden J, Carnes BA, Brody J, Hayflick L, Butler RN, Allison DB, Ludwig DS. A Potential Decline in Life Expectancy in the United States in the 21st Century. *N Engl J Med* 2005;352(11):1138–45.

Paolisso G, Ammendola S, Del Buono A, Gambardella A, Riondino M, Tagliamonte MR, Rizzo MR, Carella C, Varricchio M. Serum Levels of Insulin-Like Growth Factor-I (IGF-I) and IGF-Binding Protein-3 in Healthy Centenarians: Relationship with Plasma Leptin and Lipid Concentrations, Insulin Action, and Cognitive Function. *J Clin Endocrinol Metab* 1997;82(7):2204–9.

Paolisso G, D'Amore A, Giugliano D, Ceriello A, Varricchio M, D'Onofrio F. Pharmacologic Doses of Vitamin E Improve Insulin Action in Healthy Subjects and Non-Insulin-Dependent Diabetic Patients. *Am J Clin Nutr* 1993;57(5):650–6.

Plantinga LC, Crews DC, Coresh J, Miller ER 3rd, Saran R, Yee J, Hedgeman E, Pavkov M, Eberhardt MS, Williams DE, Powe NR. Prevalence of Chronic Kidney Disease in US Adults with Undiagnosed Diabetes or Prediabetes. *Clin J Am Soc Nephrol* 2010;5(4):673–82.

Sanyal AJ, Chalasani N, Kowdley KV, McCullough A, Diehl AM, Bass NM, Neuschwander-Tetri BA, Lavine JE, Tonascia J, Unalp A, Van Natta M, Clark J, Brunt EM, Kleiner DE, Hoofnagle JH, Robuck PR. Pioglitazone, Vitamin E, or Placebo for Nonalcoholic Steatohepatitis. *N Engl J Med* 2010;362(18):1675–85.

Selvin E, Steffes MW, Zhu H, Matsushita K, Wagenknecht L, Pankow J, Coresh J, Brancati FL. Glycated Hemoglobin, Diabetes, and Cardiovascular Risk in Nondiabetic Adults. *N Engl J Med* 2010;362(9):800–11.

Taylor SE, Klein LC, Lewis BP, Gruenewald TL, Gurung RA, Updegraff JA. Biobehavioral Responses to Stress in Females: Tend-and-Befriend, Not Fight-Or-Flight. *Psychol Rev* 2000;107(3):411–29.

US Department of Health and Human Services. Polycystic Ovary Syndrome (PCOS): Frequently Asked Questions. Womenshealth.gov, March 17, 2010. http://www.womenshealth.gov/faq/polycystic-ovary-syndrome.cfm.

Yaffe K, Weston AL, Blackwell T, Krueger KA. The Metabolic Syndrome and Development of Cognitive Impairment among Older Women. *Arch Neurol* 2009;66(3):324–8.

Chapter Eight

Adams KF, Schatzkin A, Harris TB, Kipnis V, Mouw T, Ballard-Barbash R, Hollenbeck A, Leitzmann MF. Overweight, Obesity, and Mortality in a Large Prospective Cohort of Persons 50 to 71 Years Old. *N Engl J Med* 2006;355(8):763–78.

Alley DE, Chang VW. Metabolic Syndrome and Weight Gain in Adulthood. *J Gerontol A Biol Sci Med Sci* 2010;65A(1):111–7.

Barceló A, Barbé F, Llompart E, de la Peña M, Durán-Cantolla J, Ladaria A, Bosch M, Guerra L, Agustí AG. Neuropeptide Y and Leptin in Patients with Obstructive Sleep Apnea Syndrome: Role of Obesity. *Am J Respir Crit Care Med* 2005;171(2):183–7.

Bates T, Albright J, Andersen K, Beth D, Dunn C, Ezzell J, Schneider L, Sullivan C, Vodicka S. Re-Think Your Drink. North Carolina Cooperative Extension, February 2008. http://www.ces.ncsu.edu/depts/fcs/pdfs/RethinkDrink_School_Age.pdf.

Bray GA, Nielsen SJ, Popkin BM. Consumption of High-Fructose Corn Syrup in Beverages May Play a Role in the Epidemic of Obesity. *Am J Clin Nutr* 2004;79(4):537–43.

Cappuccio FP, D'Elia L, Strazzullo P, Miller MA. Sleep Duration and All-Cause Mortality: A Systematic Review and Meta-Analysis of Prospective Studies. *Sleep* 2010;33(5):585–92.

Dhingra R, Sullivan L, Jacques PF, Wang TJ, Fox CS, Meigs JB, D'Agostino RB, Gaziano JM, Vasan RS. Soft Drink Consumption and Risk of Developing Cardiometabolic Risk Factors and the Metabolic Syndrome in Middle-Aged Adults in the Community. *Circulation* 2007;116(5):480–8.

Djuric Z, Ellsworth JS, Ren J, Sen A, Ruffin MT. A Randomized Feasibility Trial of Brief Telephone Counseling to Increase Fruit and Vegetable Intakes. *Prev Med* 2010;50(5–6):265–71 [Epub ahead of print].

Edgar WM. Sugar Substitutes, Chewing Gum and Dental Caries—A Review. *Br Dent J* 1998;184(1):29–32.

Ensrud KE, Ewing SK, Stone KL, Cauley JA, Bowman PJ, Cummings SR. Intentional and Unintentional Weight Loss Increase Bone Loss and Hip Fracture Risk in Older Women. *J Am Geriatr Soc* 2003;51(12):1740–7.

Farah H, Buzby J. U.S. Food Consumption Up 16 Percent Since 1970. *Amber Waves*, December 2005. http://www.ers.usda.gov/AmberWaves/November05/Findings/USFoodConsumption.htm.

Flegal KM, Carroll MD, Ogden CL, Johnson CL. Prevalence and Trends in Obesity among US Adults, 1999–2000. *JAMA* 2002;288(14):1723–7.

Flegal KM, Graubard BI, Williamson DF, Gail MH. Excess Deaths Associated with Underweight, Overweight, and Obesity. *JAMA* 2005;293(15):1861–7.

Hamilton MT, Hamilton DG, Zderic TW. Role of Low Energy Expenditure and Sitting in Obesity, Metabolic Syndrome, Type 2 Diabetes, and Cardiovascular Disease. *Diabetes* 2007;56(11):2655–67.

Houston TK, Person SD, Pletcher MJ, Liu K, Iribarren C, Kiefe CI. Active and Passive Smoking and Development of Glucose Intolerance among Young Adults in a Prospective Cohort: CARDIA Study. *BMJ* 2006;332(7549):1064–9.

Karuppagounder SS, Pinto JT, Xu H, Chen HL, Beal MF, Gibson GE. Dietary Supplementation with Resveratrol Reduces Plaque Pathology in a Transgenic Model of Alzheimer's Disease. *Neurochem Int* 2009;54(2):111–8.

Lee JM, Pilli S, Gebremariam A, Keirns CC, Davis MM, Vijan S, Freed GL, Herman WH, Gurney JG. Getting Heavier, Younger: Trajectories of Obesity over the Life Course. *Int J Obes (Lond)* 2010;34(4):61423.

Levine J, Baukol P, Pavlidis I. The Energy Expended in Chewing Gum. *N Engl J Med* 1999;341(27):2100.

Lumeng JC, Forrest P, Appugliese DP, Kaciroti N, Corwyn RF, Bradley RH. Weight Status as a Predictor of Being Bullied in Third through Sixth Grades. *Pediatrics* May 3, 2010 [Epub ahead of print].

Ma Y, Bertone ER, Stanek EJ 3rd, Reed GW, Hebert JR, Cohen NL, Merriam PA, Ockene IS. Association between Eating Patterns and Obesity in a Free-Living US Adult Population. *Am J Epidemiol* 2003;158(1):85-92.

Maruyama K, Sato S, Ohira T, Maeda K, Noda H, Kubota Y, Nishimura S, Kitamura A, Kiyama M, Okada T, Imano H, Nakamura M, Ishikawa Y, Kurokawa M, Sasaki S, Iso H. The Joint Impact on Being Overweight of Self Reported Behaviours of Eating Quickly and Eating Until Full: Cross Sectional Survey. *BMJ* 2008;337: a2002.

McAllister EJ, Dhurandhar NV, Keith SW, Aronne LJ, Barger J, Baskin M, Benca RM, Biggio J, Boggiano MM, Eisenmann JC, Elobeid M, Fontaine KR, Gluckman P, Hanlon EC, Katzmarzyk P, Pietrobelli A, Redden DT, Ruden DM, Wang C, Waterland RA, Wright SM, Allison DB. Ten Putative Contributors to the Obesity Epidemic. *Crit Rev Food Sci Nutr* 2009;49(10):868–913.

McCarty CA, McCarty DJ, Wetter AC. Calories from Newspaper Dessert Recipes Are Associated with Community Obesity Rates. *WMJ* 2007;106(2):68–70.

Mummery WK, Schofield GM, Steele R, Eakin EG, Brown WJ. Occupational Sitting Time and Overweight and Obesity in Australian Workers. *Am J Prev Med* 2005;29(2):91–7.

National Institute of Diabetes and Digestive and Kidney Diseases, National Institutes of Health. Statistics Related to Overweight and Obesity. Weight-Control Information Network, February 2010. http://www.win.niddk.nih.gov/statistics/index.htm.

Newsom SA, Schenk S, Thomas KM, Harber MP, Knuth ND, Goldenberg N, Horowitz JF. Energy Deficit after Exercise Augments Lipid Mobilization but Does Not Contribute to the Exercise-Induced Increase in Insulin Sensitivity. *J Appl Physiol* 2010;108(3):554–60.

O'Brien PE, McPhail T, Chaston TB, Dixon JB. Systematic Review of Medium-Term Weight Loss after Bariatric Operations. *Obes Surg* 2006;16(6):1032–40.

Olshansky SJ, Passaro DJ, Hershow RC, Layden J, Carnes BA, Brody J, Hayflick L, Butler RN, Allison DB, Ludwig DS. A Potential Decline in Life Expectancy in the United States in the 21st Century. *N Engl J Med* 2005;352(11):1138–45.

Putnam JJ, Allshouse JE. Food Consumption, Prices, and Expenditures, 1970–97. Statistical Bulletin No. SB-965. Washington, DC: Economic Research Service, US Department of Agriculture, 1999.

Rajaratnam JK, Marcus JR, Levin-Rector A, Chalupka AN, Wang H, Dwyer L, Costa M, Lopez AD, Murray CJ. Worldwide Mortality in Men and Women Aged 15–59 Years from 1970 to 2010: A Systematic Analysis. *Lancet* 2010;375(9727):1704–20.

Raji CA, Ho AJ, Parikshak NN, Becker JT, Lopez OL, Kuller LH, Hua X, Leow AD, Toga AW, Thompson PM. Brain Structure and Obesity. *Hum Brain Mapp* 2010;31(3):353–64.

Singh GK, Kogan MD, van Dyck PC. Changes in State-Specific Childhood Obesity and Overweight Prevalence in the United States from 2003 to 2007. *Arch Pediatr Adolesc Med* 2010;164(7) [Epub ahead of print].

Singh GK, Siahpush M, Kogan MD. Neighborhood Socioeconomic Conditions, Built Environments, and Childhood Obesity. *Health Aff (Millwood)* 2010;29(3):503–12.

Slentz CA, Aiken LB, Houmard JA, Bales CW, Johnson JL, Tanner CJ, Duscha BD, Kraus WE. Inactivity, Exercise, and Visceral Fat. STRRIDE: A Randomized, Controlled Study of Exercise Intensity and Amount. *J Appl Physiol* 2005;99(4):1613–8.

University of California, San Francisco, Medical Center. Bariatric Surgery. March 30, 2010. http://www.ucsfhealth.org/adult/medical_services/gastro/bariatric/conditions/surgery/treatments.html.

Vartanian LR, Schwartz MB, Brownell KD. Effects of Soft Drink Consumption on Nutrition and Health: A Systematic Review and Meta-Analysis. *Am J Public Health* 2007;97(4):667–75.

Vgontzas AN, Papanicolaou DA, Bixler EO, Hopper K, Lotsikas A, Lin HM, Kales A, Chrousos GP. Sleep Apnea and Daytime Sleepiness and Fatigue: Relation to Visceral Obesity, Insulin Resistance, and Hypercytokinemia. *J Clin Endocrinol Metab* 2000;85(3):1151–8.

Wang L, Lee IM, Manson JE, Buring JE, Sesso HD. Alcohol Consumption, Weight Gain, and Risk of Becoming Overweight in Middle-Aged and Older Women. *Arch Intern Med* 2010;170(5):453–61.

Wittgrove AC, Clark GW, Schubert KR. Laparoscopic Gastric Bypass, Roux-en-Y: Technique and Results in 75 Patients with 3-30 Months Follow-Up. *Obes Surg* 1996;6(6):500–4.

Zhong CB, DeVoe SE. You Are How You Eat: Fast Food and Impatience. *Psychol Sci* 2010;5:619–22.

Chapter Nine

Barton J, Pretty J. What Is the Best Dose of Nature and Green Exercise for Improving Mental Health? A Multi-Study Analysis. *Environ Sci Technol* 2010;44(10):3947–55.

Brummett BH, Boyle SH, Ortel TL, Becker RC, Siegler IC, Williams RB. Associations of Depressive Symptoms, Trait Hostility, and Gender with C-Reactive Protein and Interleukin-6 Response after Emotion Recall. *Psychosom Med* 2010;72(4):333–9.

Christakis NA, Fowler JH. The Spread of Obesity in a Large Social Network over 32 Years. *N Engl J Med* 2007;357(4):370–9.

Christenfeld N, Gerin W, Linden W, Sanders M, Mathur J, Deich JD, Pickering TG. Social Support Effects on Cardiovascular Reactivity: Is a Stranger as Effective as a Friend? *Psychosom Med* 1997;59(4):388–98.

Crusco AH, Wetzel CG. The Midas Touch. *Pers Soc Psychol Bull* 1984;10(4):512–7.

Davidson KW, Mostofsky E. Anger Expression and Risk of Coronary Heart Disease: Evidence from the Nova Scotia Health Survey. *Am Heart J* 2010;159(2):199–206.

Fowler JH, Christakis NA. Dynamic Spread of Happiness in a Large Social Network: Longitudinal Analysis over 20 Years in the Framingham Heart Study. *BMJ* 2008;337:a2338.

Fowler JH, Christakis NA. Cooperative Behavior Cascades in Human Social Networks. *Proc Natl Acad Sci U S A* 2010;107(12):5334–8.

Hertenstein MJ, Holmes R, McCullough M, Keltner D. The Communication of Emotion via Touch. *Emotion* 2009;9(4):566–73.

Hughes ME, Waite LJ. Marital Biography and Health at Mid-Life. *J Health Soc Behav* 2009;50(3):344–58.

Keller MC, Fredrickson BL, Ybarra O, Côté S, Johnson K, Mikels J, Conway A, Wager T. A Warm Heart and a Clear Head. The Contingent Effects of Weather on Mood and Cognition. *Psychol Sci* 2005;16(9):724–31.

Lambert NM, Fincham FD, Stillman TF, Graham SM, Beach SR. Motivating Change in Relationships: Can Prayer Increase Forgiveness? *Psychol Sci* 2010;21(1):126–32.

Lemogne C, Nabi H, Zins M, Cordier S, Ducimetière P, Goldberg M, Consoli SM. Hostility May Explain the Association between Depressive Mood and Mortality: Evidence from the French GAZEL Cohort Study. *Psychother Psychosom* 2010;79(3):164–171.

Lewis TT, Everson-Rose SA, Karavolos K, Janssen I, Wesley D, Powell LH. Hostility Is Associated with Visceral, but Not Subcutaneous, Fat in Middle-Aged African American and White Women. *Psychosom Med* 2009;71(7):733–40.

Little JT, Reynolds CF 3rd, Dew MA, Frank E, Begley AE, Miller MD, Cornes C, Mazumdar S, Perel JM, Kupfer DJ. How Common Is Resistance to Treatment in Recurrent, Nonpsychotic Geriatric Depression? *Am J Psychiatry* 1998;155(8):1035–8.

Mednick SC, Christakis NA, Fowler JH. The Spread of Sleep Loss Influences Drug Use in Adolescent Social Networks. *PLoS ONE* 2010;5(3):e9775.

Mezick EJ, Matthews KA, Hall M, Kamarck TW, Strollo PJ, Buysse DJ, Owens JF, Reis SE. Low Life Purpose and High Hostility Are Related to an Attenuated Decline in Nocturnal Blood Pressure. *Health Psychol* 2010;29(2):196–204.

Newsom JT, Schulz R. Social Support as a Mediator in the Relation between Functional Status and Quality of Life in Older Adults. *Psychol Aging* 1996;11(1):34–44.

Otake K, Shimai S, Tanaka-Matsumi J, Otsui K, Fredrickson BL. Happy People Become Happier through Kindness: A Counting Kindnesses Intervention. *J Happiness Stud* 2006;7(3):361–75.

Paul CL, Ross S, Bryant J, Hill W, Bonevski B, Keevy N. The Social Context of Smoking: A Qualitative Study Comparing Smokers of High versus Low Socioeconomic Position. *BMC Public Health* 2010;10(1):211.

Richter M, Eck J, Straube T, Miltner WH, Weiss T. Do Words Hurt? Brain Activation during the Processing of Pain-Related Words. *Pain* 2010;148(2):198–205.

Saxbe D, Repetti RL. For Better or Worse? Coregulation of Couples' Cortisol Levels and Mood States. *J Pers Soc Psychol* 2010;98(1):92–103.

Chapter Ten

Agency for Health Care Research and Quality. Overview: Urinary Incontinence in Adults: Clinical Practice Guideline Update. March 1996. http://www.ahrq.gov/clinic/uiovervw.htm.

Diego MA, Jones NA, Field T, Hernandez-Reif M, Schanberg S, Kuhn C, Gonzalez-Garcia A. Maternal Psychological Distress, Prenatal Cortisol, and Fetal Weight. *Psychosom Med* 2006;68(5):747–53.

Evenson KR, Wen F. National Trends in Self-Reported Physical Activity and Sedentary Behaviors among Pregnant Women: NHANES 1999–2006. *Prev Med* 2010;50(3):123–8.

Field T, Figueiredo B, Hernandez-Reif M, Diego M, Deeds O, Ascencio A, Bodyw J. Massage Therapy Reduces Pain in Pregnant Women, Alleviates Prenatal Depression in Both Parents and Improves Their Relationships. *Mov Ther* 2008;12(2):146–50.

Foxman B, Barlow R, D'Arcy H, Gillespie B, Sobel JD. Urinary Tract Infection: Self-Reported Incidence and Associated Costs. *Ann Epidemiol* 2000;10(8):509–15.

Greening DJ. Frequent Ejaculation. A Pilot Study of Changes in Sperm DNA Damage and Semen Parameters Using Daily Ejaculation. *Fertil Steril* 2007;88 Suppl 1:S19–20.

Hall SA, Shackelton R, Rosen RC, Araujo AB. Sexual Activity, Erectile Dysfunction, and Incident Cardiovascular Events. *Am J Cardiol* 2010;105(2):192–7.

Marshall AM, Nommsen-Rivers LA, Hernandez LL, Dewey KG, Chantry CJ, Gregerson KA, Horseman ND. Serotonin Transport and Metabolism in the Mammary Gland Modulates Secretory Activation and Involution. *J Clin Endocrinol Metab* 2010;95(2):837–46.

Söder B, Yakob M, Nowak J, Jogestrand T. Risk for the Development of Atherosclerosis in Women with a High Amount [Corrected] of Dental Plaque and Severe Gingival Inflammation. *Int J Dent Hyg* 2007;5(3):133–8.

Swanson MD, Winter HC, Goldstein IJ, Markovitz DM. A Lectin Isolated from Bananas is a Potent Inhibitor of HIV Replication. *J Biol Chem* 2010;285(12):8646–55.

University of Maryland Medical Center. Pregnancy Guide: Genetic Counseling. n.d. http://www.umm.edu/pregnancy/000092.htm.

Vine MF. Smoking and Male Reproduction: A Review. *Int J Androl* 1996;19(6):323–37.

Chapter Eleven

Arenz S, Rückerl R, Koletzko B, von Kries R. Breast-Feeding and Childhood Obesity—A Systematic Review. *Int J Obes Relat Metab Disord* 2004;28(10):1247–56.

Bhattacharyya N, Shapiro NL. Air Quality Improvement and the Prevalence of Frequent Ear Infections in Children. *Otolaryngol Head Neck Surg* 2010;142(2):242–6.

Dawson G, Rogers S, Munson J, Smith M, Winter J, Greenson J, Donaldson A, Varley J. Randomized, Controlled Trial of an Intervention for Toddlers with Autism: The Early Start Denver Model. *Pediatrics* 2010;125(1):e17–23.

Fors S, Lennartsson C, Lundberg O. Childhood Living Conditions, Socioeconomic Position in Adulthood, and Cognition in Later Life: Exploring the Associations. *Gerontol B Psychol Sci Soc Sci* 2009;64(6):750–7.

Gordon I, Zagoory-Sharon O, Leckman JF, Feldman R. Oxytocin and the Development of Parenting in Humans. *Biol Psychiatry* Apr 1, 2010 [Epub ahead of print].

Herman KM, Craig CL, Gauvin L, Katzmarzyk PT. Tracking of Obesity and Physical Activity from Childhood to Adulthood: The Physical Activity Longitudinal Study. *Int J Pediatr Obes* 2009;4(4):281–8.

Hunziker UA, Barr RG. Increased Carrying Reduces Infant Crying: A Randomized Controlled Trial. *Pediatrics* 1986;77(5):641–8.

Kemp JS, Unger B, Wilkins D, Psara RM, Ledbetter TL, Graham MA, Case M, Thach BT. Unsafe Sleep Practices and an Analysis of Bedsharing among Infants Dying Suddenly and Unexpectedly: Results of a Four-Year, Population-Based, Death-Scene Investigation Study of Sudden Infant Death Syndrome and Related Deaths. *Pediatrics* 2000;106(3):E41.

Lai HL, Chen CJ, Peng TC, Chang FM, Hsieh ML, Huang HY, Chang SC. Randomized Controlled Trial of Music During Kangaroo Care on Maternal State Anxiety and Preterm Infants' Responses. *Int J Nurs Stud* 2006;43(2):139–46.

Liu B, Jorm L, Banks E. Parity, Breastfeeding and the Subsequent Risk of Maternal Type 2 Diabetes. *Diabetes Care* Mar 23, 2010 [Epub ahead of print].

McConnell R, Islam T, Shankardass K, Jerrett M, Lurmann F, Gilliland F, Gauderman J, Avol E, Kuenzli N, Yao L, Peters J, Berhane K. Childhood Incident Asthma and Traffic-Related Air Pollution at Home and School. *Environ Health Perspect* Mar 22, 2010 [Epub ahead of print].

Nakamura S, Wind M, Danello MA. Review of Hazards Associated with Children Placed in Adult Beds. *Arch Pediatr Adolesc Med* 1999;153(10):1019–23.

Nwosu BU, Lee MM. Evaluation of Short and Tall Stature in Children. *Am Fam Physician* 2008;78(5):597–604.

Nyqvist KH, Anderson GC, Bergman N, Cattaneo A, Charpak N, Davanzo R, Ewald U, Ibe O, Ludington-Hoe S, Mendoza S, Pallás-Allonso C, Peláez JG, Sizun J, Widström AM. Towards Universal Kangaroo Mother Care: Recommendations and Report from the First European Conference and Seventh International Workshop on Kangaroo Mother Care. *Acta Paediatr* 2010;99(6):820–6.

Okami P, Weisner T, Olmstead R. Outcome Correlates of Parent-Child Bedsharing: An Eighteen-Year Longitudinal Study. *J Dev Behav Pediatr* 2002;23(4):244–53.

Piernas C, Popkin BM. Trends in Snacking among U.S. Children. *Health Aff (Millwood)* 2010;29(3):398–404.

Preston SH, Hill ME, Drevenstedt GL. Childhood Conditions That Predict Survival to Advanced Ages among African-Americans. *Soc Sci Med* 1998;47(9):1231–46.

Schack-Nielsen L, Michaelsen KF. Breast Feeding and Future Health. *Curr Opin Clin Nutr Metab Care* 2006;9(3):289–96.

Shah SS, Wood SM, Luan X, Ratner AJ. Decline in Varicella-Related Ambulatory Visits and Hospitalizations in the United States Since Routine Immunization Against Varicella. *Pediatr Infect Dis J* 2010;29(3):199–204.

Slining M, Adair LS, Goldman BD, Borja JB, Bentley M. Infant Overweight Is Associated with Delayed Motor Development. *J Pediatr* Mar 12, 2010 [Epub ahead of print].

Stuebe AM, Michels KB, Willett WC, Manson JE, Rexrode K, Rich-Edwards JW. Duration of Lactation and Incidence of Myocardial Infarction in Middle to Late Adulthood. *Am J Obstet Gynecol* 2009;200(2):138.e1–8.

Stuebe AM, Rich-Edwards JW, Willett WC, Manson JE, Michels KB. Duration of Lactation and Incidence of Type 2 Diabetes. *JAMA* 2005;294(20):2601–10.

Taylor CA, Manganello JA, Lee SJ, Rice JC. Mothers' Spanking of 3-Year-Old Children and Subsequent Risk of Children's Aggressive Behavior. *Pediatrics* 2010;125(5):e1057–65.

Uvnäs-Moberg K, Widström AM, Werner S, Matthiesen AS, Winberg J. Oxytocin and Prolactin Levels in Breast-Feeding Women. Correlation with Milk Yield and Duration of Breast-Feeding. *Acta Obstet Gynecol Scand* 1990;69(4):301–6.

About the
Doctors

Travis Stork, MD

When he isn't hosting the syndicated series, Dr. Stork is a faculty physician in the Emergency Department at Vanderbilt Medical Center in Nashville, Tennessee.

His credentials include graduating magna cum laude from Duke University and earning his MD with honors from the University of Virginia. He completed his residency as an emergency room doctor at Vanderbilt University.

Dr. Stork writes a monthly column for *Men's Health* magazine and recently wrote a book called *The Doctor Is In,* which teaches readers how simple changes now may add quality years to their lives later.

An avid outdoorsman, Dr. Stork is a devotee of mountain and road biking, kayaking, and hiking with his dog, Nala.

Lisa M. Masterson, MD

Dr. Masterson is a specialist in obstetrics, gynecology, infertility, adolescent gynecology, and family planning. She is on staff at Los Angeles's Cedars-Sinai Medical Center, St. John's Hospital in Santa Monica, and UCLA, and maintains a private practice in Santa Monica.

Dr. Masterson is a founder and medical director of the Ocean Oasis Medical Spa in Santa Monica, which offers spa treatments and exercise and nutrition programs tailored specifically for women. She attended the Bishop's School, a private school in La Jolla, California, and upon graduation, entered Mount Holyoke College in Massachusetts. She graduated from medical school at the University of Southern California.

In 2008, Dr. Masterson received the Golden Rattle Award from the March of Dimes in recognition of her advocacy for improving the health of babies and mothers all over the world. In 2007, she received the Red Cross Humanitarian Award. Her groundbreaking research was published in the journal *Obstetrics & Gynecology* in 1994.

Dr. Masterson's memoir, *Paper Dollhouse,* will be published by Globe Pequot in 2011. She has a son and lives in Southern California. In her spare time, she enjoys surfing and learning French.

James M. Sears, MD

Dr. James (Jim) is a board-certified pediatrician who is part of a family practice that he shares with his father, William, and younger brother Robert, located in Capistrano Beach, California.

He earned his medical degree at St. Louis University School of Medicine in 1996 and completed his pediatric residency at Northeastern Ohio University College of Medicine and Tod Children's Hospital in Youngstown, Ohio, in 1999. During his residency, he received the honor of "Emergency Medicine Resident of the Year."

Dr. Sears currently serves as a regular contributor for AOLHealth.com. He has coauthored several books, including *The Healthiest Kid in the Neighborhood, Father's First Steps, The Premature Baby Book, The Baby Sleep Book,* and the best-selling *The Baby Book.*

A father of two, his personal passions include endurance cycling, mountain biking, triathlons, sailboat racing, snow skiing, hiking, and acting in musical theater with his daughter.

Andrew P. Ordon, MD, FACS

For over two decades, Dr. Ordon has been an acclaimed surgeon in the area of aesthetic plastic and reconstructive surgery with a private practice in New York City and now in Beverly Hills and Rancho Mirage, California. He is the author of *Revealing the New You* and *Everything You Always Wanted to Know about Plastic Surgery* and contributed to one of the best textbooks in the field of plastic surgery, *Facial Aesthetic Plastic Surgery.*

One of Dr. Ordon's proudest accomplishments has been as a founding member of the Surgical Friends Foundation (www.surgicalfriends.org). Surgical Friends is comprised of a group of doctors who offer complimentary reconstructive surgery to those both domestically and abroad who otherwise could not afford medical treatment. Many of these patients have suffered from birth defects, physical abuse, and burns among other adverse conditions.

Dr. Ordon is a Phi Beta Kappa graduate of the University of California, Irvine, with a medical degree from the USC School of Medicine with honors. His general surgery and head and neck surgery training were completed at USC, UCLA, and Loma Linda, respectively. He then completed his training program in plastic and reconstructive surgery at the Lenox Hill Hospital/Manhattan Eye and Ear Infirmary Program.

Dr. Ordon is currently an assistant clinical professor of plastic surgery at Dartmouth Medical College and the UCLA School of Medicine. He is a member of the American Society of Plastic Surgeons, the American Society for Aesthetic Plastic Surgery, the International Society for Aesthetic Plastic Surgery, the Double Boarded Society of Plastic Surgeons and the California Society of Plastic Surgeons. In addition, he is a Diplomate with the American Board of Plastic Surgery, the American Board of Otolaryngology & Head and Neck Surgery, the American Board of Cosmetic Surgery, and the National Board of Medical Examiners. He is a Fellow with the American College of Surgeons, the International College of Surgeons, and the American Academy of Facial Plastic and Reconstructive Surgery.

Born and raised in Long Beach, California, Dr. Ordon and his wife, a former Wilhelmina model turned interior designer, live in West Hollywood and Rancho Mirage. They have two children who are presently attending college. In his spare time, Dr. Ordon enjoys surfing, skiing, golf, and tennis.

Index

Boldface page references indicate illustrations. <u>Underscored</u> page references indicate boxed text.

A

ABCDs of mole exams, 138–39
Abdominal pain, <u>98–99</u>
Acceptance, 207–8
Acetaminophen, <u>160</u>
Acid-stopping proton pump inhibitors, <u>91</u>
Acne, 140–41
Acuflex, 293
Additives, food, 104
ADHD, 109–10
Adrenal glands, 154
Adrenaline, 161
AED (automated external defibrillator) and training, 36, <u>37</u>
Aerobic exercise, 57, 193
Aging
    brain and, 48–49
    exceptional, 5–6, 49
    fish oil supplements in managing, <u>30</u>
    hormones and, 144, 163–65
    musculoskeletal system and, 119–20
    skin and, 119–20
    weight and, 189
Air conditioner, turning down, 193
Air fresheners, avoiding, 80
Air swallowing, 94
Alcohol, 29, 32, <u>111</u>, 190, 192. *See also specific type*
Aldosterone, 154
Allergies, 67, <u>71</u>, 74, 80–81, 268, <u>275</u>
Almonds, <u>101</u>
Aloe vera, 132–33, <u>133</u>
Alveoli, 68
Alzheimer's disease, 48, <u>56</u>, 58, 61. *See also* Cognitive decline
Androgens, <u>159</u>, 161
Androsterone, 236
Anger, <u>217</u>
Anticipation, 25–26
Anxiety, social, <u>206</u>
Appendicitis, <u>98</u>
Appetite suppressant, 193
Apple cider vinegar, 173–74
Apples, 9, 35, <u>101</u>
Aromatase, <u>160</u>
Arrhythmia, 28, <u>37</u>

Arteries, clogged, 18–19, 36–37
Arthritis, 120, 123
Aspirin, 53, <u>160</u>
Asthma, 69, <u>70</u>, 76, 272, <u>275</u>
Atherosclerosis, 19
Autism, <u>276–77</u>
Avocados, 236

B

Bamboo charcoal filters, 80
Bananas, 56–57
BanLec, <u>230</u>
Barefoot walking, <u>145</u>
Bariatric surgery, <u>188–89</u>
Beano, <u>95</u>
Beans, <u>95</u>
Beef, 74
Beer, 29
Belly fat, 158, 160
Beverages. *See specific type*
Bioidentical hormones, <u>168–69</u>
Bisphenol A (BPA), 76, 78, 135, <u>167</u>
Blackheads, 140
Bladder infection, 242
Bleeding, <u>47</u>. *See also* Menstruation
Blood pressure, 20, 22, <u>23</u>, 29, 37, 164. *See also* High blood pressure
Blood sugar levels, 26, 37, 154, <u>164</u>, 165–66, 173
Blood sugar tests, 173, 291, <u>291</u>
Blood tests, 26, 173, <u>291</u>, 292
Blood vessels, 17, <u>47</u>
Blueberries, <u>281</u>
Blue vegetables, 113
BMI, <u>167</u>, 183–84, 288
Body fat, 63, 152, 158, 160, 204
Body image, <u>210–11</u>
Body mass index (BMI), <u>167</u>, 183–84, 288
Bone density scan, <u>129</u>
Bones, 120–22, 153, 189. *See also* Musculoskeletal system
Botox, <u>142–43</u>
Bottle feeding, 268
Boundaries, healthy personal, 207–8
Bowel movements, <u>112</u>, <u>114–15</u>, <u>243</u>, 265

BPA, 76, 78, 135, <u>167</u>
Brain
    aging and, 48–49
    anatomy, 42
    cognitive decline and, 43, 56, <u>164</u>
    complexity of, 42–43
    cortisol and, 44
    development of, 46–48
    dietary fat and, 43
    evolution and, 41
    health fixes for
        aspirin, 53
        breathing, deep, 55
        chewing gum, 49
        clutter, reducing, 62
        computer, using, 5
        diet, 43, 49–50, 53–54, 56–59
        exercise, 52–53, 55–59
        fish, smoked, 49–50
        five tips, <u>41</u>
        helmets, 45
        hygiene, practicing good, 61–62
        mindfulness meditation, <u>50–51</u>
        napping, 50–52
        sleep, 44, 50–52, 63
        standing, 54–55
        waistline measurement, reducing, <u>60–61</u>
        yoga, 57–58
    high blood pressure and, 56–57
    importance of, 41
    infections and, 61–62
    injuries, 45, <u>46–47</u>
    left side, 42
    longevity and healthy, 6
    neuron connections, 46–48
    pregnancy and, <u>249</u>
    protecting, 45, 120
    right side, 42
    sleep and, 44, 63
    stroke and, <u>45</u>
    waistline measurement and, <u>60–61</u>
Bread crumbs substitution, 32
Breastfeeding, 262, 264–65, 268, 270
Breast cancer, <u>160</u>

Crohn's disease, <u>115</u>
Croup, <u>71</u>
CRP, 22, 53
Cuddling, 265–66
Curcumin, <u>33</u>
Cycling, 55–56
Cytokines, 58

D

d-alpha tocopherol, 170
DASH (Dietary Approaches to Stop Hypertension) diet, 32, 57
Day care, selecting, 272–73
Decongestants, <u>75</u>
Deep breathing techniques, 55
Dehydration, <u>106</u>, <u>131</u>
Dehydroepiandrosterone (DHEA), 154
Dementia, 43, 56. *See also* Alzheimer's disease
Denial of health problems, 26, 279
Dental health fixes, 134–35, 248–50, 268
Depression, <u>212–13</u>
Dermis, 124
DHA, <u>30</u>, 53
DHEA, 154
Diabetes, 5, <u>130</u>, 152, <u>156</u>, 170, 173. *See also* Type 1 diabetes; Type 2 diabetes
Diagnostic tests. *See* Tests
Diaper rash cream, 132–33
Diaphragm, 68
Diarrhea, <u>103</u>, <u>114</u>
Diastolic pressure, 20, <u>23</u>
Diet. *See also* Food
    DASH, 32, 57
    digestive system and, 87, 90, 93–94
    fever and, <u>79</u>
    as health fix for
        brain, 43, 49–50, 53–54, 56–59
        childhood years, 270–71, 275–78
        digestive system, <u>91</u>, 100, <u>101</u>, 102–4, <u>103</u>, 107–10
        heart, 26–27, 32–33
        lungs, 73–74
        pregnancy, 246–47
        reproductive system, 236
        weight, 193, <u>195</u>, <u>196</u>, 197

high-fiber, 94–95
modern, 43
nutrient-dense, 100, 112
in preventing
    gastroesophageal reflux disease, <u>91</u>
    heartburn, <u>91</u>
    high blood pressure, 32, 57
Dietary fat, 43, 100. *See also specific type*
Dieting, <u>196</u>
Diet soda, 106
Digestion, 7, 92–94
Digestive problems. *See specific type*
Digestive system
    abdominal pain and, <u>98–99</u>
    anatomy, 92
    bowel movements and, <u>112</u>, <u>114–15</u>
    diet and, 87, 90, 93–94
    gas and, 94–96, <u>95</u>
    health fixes for
        alcohol intake, reducing, <u>111</u>
        diet, <u>91</u>, 100, <u>101</u>, 102–4, <u>103</u>, 107–10
        five tips, <u>87</u>
        green tea, 110
        homemade lunches, 110–11
        probiotics, 102–4
        soda, avoiding, 104–7
        water intake, <u>106–7</u>
    importance of, 87
    longevity and healthy, 7
    pathogens and, 96–97, 100
    stomach acid and, <u>91</u>
    urine color and, <u>115</u>
Dihydrocapsiate, <u>194</u>
Disciplinary techniques for children, 273–75
Docosahexaenoic acid (DHA), <u>30</u>, 53
Dose response effect, 215
Dressings, salad, 58–59
Driving, 9
Drugs. *See* Medications; *specific type*
Dumbbells, 147

E

Ear infections, 272
ED, 34, <u>239</u>

Eggs, 170–72
Eicosapentaenoic acid (EPA), <u>30</u>, 53
Elance.com, 196
Emergency Cardiovascular Care (ECC) Class Connector, 36
Emotional health, 203–4
Endocrine disruptors, 151
Endocrine essay, 173
Endocrine system
    anatomy, 152–55
    disruptors, 151
    energy and, 158–61
    function of, 151
    health fixes for
        apple cider vinegar, 173–74
        brown rice, 166
        chemical toxins, avoiding, 174–76
        cinnamon, 173–74
        diabetes medications, avoiding, 165–66
        eggs, 170–72
        fast food, avoiding, 170
        five tips, 152
        hormone screen, 173
        laughter, 172
        vitamin E, 166, 168–70
    interconnectedness of, 164
    longevity and healthy, 7
    stress and, 160–61
Endorphins, 153, 236
Energy, 90, 158–61
Enzyme deficiency, 123
EPA, <u>30</u>, 53
Epidermis, 124
Epinephrine, 154, 160
Erectile dysfunction (ED), 34, <u>239</u>
Erections, 34
Essential fatty acids, <u>30</u>, 43, 53
Estrogen, 151, 154–55, <u>160</u>, 161, <u>168</u>, 231, <u>245</u>
Exceptional aging, 5–6, 49
Exercise. *See also specific type*
    aerobic, 57, 193
    blood pressure and, 37
    as health fix for
        brain, 52–53, 55–59
        childhood obesity, <u>191</u>
        heart, 20, 28, 35–38
        lungs, 80
        musculoskeletal system, 128, <u>129</u>, 134, 143–46